FRESH & HEALTHY
DASH
DIET COOKING

Delicious Recipes for
Lowering Blood Pressure,
Losing Weight & Feeling Great

ANDREA LYNN
with Matt Kadey MSc., Rd

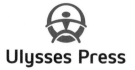

Ulysses Press

Published by
Ulysses Press
P.O. Box 3440
Berkeley, CA 94703
www.ulyssespress.com

ISBN: 978-1-61243-114-7
Library of Congress Catalog Number 2012940423

Printed in China by Everbest through Four Colour Print Group

10 9 8 7 6 5 4 3 2 1

Contributing Writer: Matt Kadey
Acquisitions Editor: Kelly Reed
Managing Editor: Claire Chun
Editor: Lauren Harrison
Production: Judith Metzener
Cover design: what!design @ whatweb.com
Photographs: © judiswinksphotography.com except on page 5 © Eric Gevaert/ fotolia.com; page 6 © Robyn Mackenzie/shutterstock.com; page 10 © Yuri Samsonov/shutterstock.com; page 11 © Charles Amundson/shutterstock.com; page 18 © Pakhnyushcha/shutterstock.com; page 28 © Yasonya/fotolia.com; page 35 © nito/shutterstock.com; page 38 © ULKASTUDIO/shutterstock .com; page 43 © Lepas/shutterstock.com; page 44 © Viktar Malyshchyts/ shutterstock.com; page 51 © xmasbaby/fotolia.com; page 79 © Nikola Bilic/ fotolia.com; page 96 © studiogi/shutterstock.com; page 109 © Evgeniy Drogozhilov/fotolia.com; page 130 © Nattika/shutterstock.com; page 135 © marekuliasz/shutterstock.com; page 137 © Nattika/shutterstock.com
Food stylist for pictured recipes: Anna Hartman-Kenzler

Distributed by Publishers Group West

Table of Contents

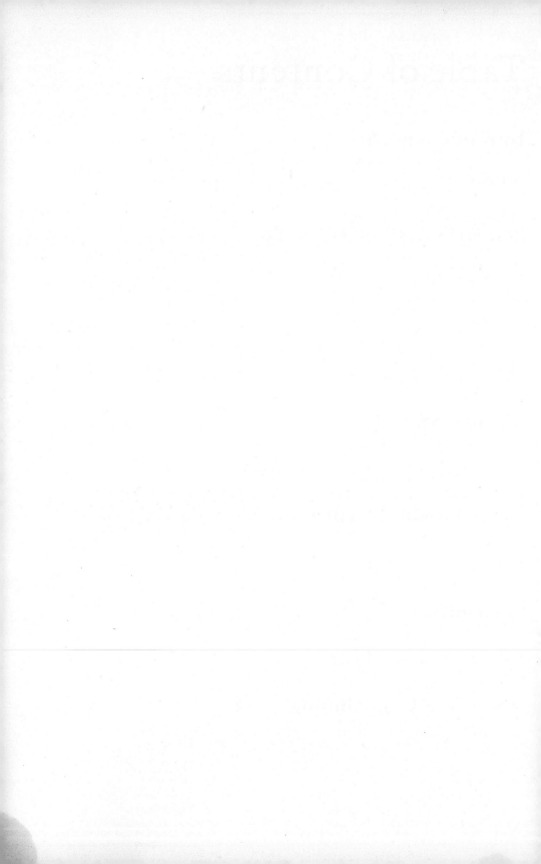

Introduction

Diet fads come and go (remember the wheat grass craze?) but the DASH Diet is definitely legit. The acronym stands for Dietary Approaches to Stop Hypertension. The plan was developed by the National Heart, Lung, and Blood Institute and involves higher intakes of whole grains, nuts, fruits, vegetables, low-fat dairy, and protein from lean sources like fish and beans, while minimizing processed grains, high-fat meats and dairy, sugars, and, of course, sodium. In other words, it's a whole-food, calorie-controlled approach to eating.

Currently, a whopping one in three American adults has hypertension, putting them at risk for heart disease, stroke, and kidney disease—leading causes of death in the U.S. According to the Centers for Disease Control and Prevention, high blood pressure was a primary or contributing cause of death for more than 347,000 Americans in 2008. What's more, nearly 30 percent of American adults have what is known as pre-hypertension, meaning their blood pressure numbers are higher than normal, but not yet in the hypertension range.

But here is the good news: Embracing the DASH Diet can help make sure that hypertension does not sour your health. An expert panel of physicians assembled by the *U.S. News & World Report* ranked the DASH Diet as the best overall diet, offering praise for its nutritional completeness, safety, and ability to fend off diseases. A raft of studies suggest that adhering to the eating patterns outlined by the DASH Diet, especially when paired with weight loss, is just as, if not more, effective at lowering blood pressure numbers than drug therapy. Investigators from New York University School of Medicine determined that the consumption of a DASH-like diet is associated with lower all-cause mortality in adults who suffer from hypertension.

The collection of recipes in this book is geared toward adhering to the primary nutritional guidelines outlined by this all-star diet. And even better, they are delicious while also being chock-full of whole, *real* foods and stripped of undesirables like salt, sugar, and saturated fat. Somehow

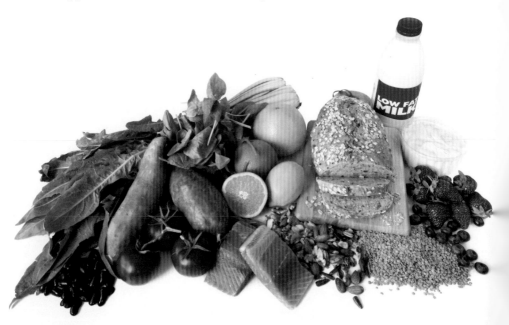

this way of eating has lost its way in America and the consequences have been clear, as obesity rates and health care costs have skyrocketed. You'll find eating a DASH-style diet to be flexible, balanced, and tasty. It's the ideal way to take back control of your health.

Do the DASH

Even if your blood pressure is perfect, there are plenty of reasons to still give the DASH Diet a shot:

- Scientists at Harvard School of Public Health discovered that eating more healthy meals that adhere to the DASH Diet guidelines can be protective against colorectal cancer—one of the leading causes of cancer-related deaths in the United States.
- A separate Harvard study indicates that following the DASH Diet can significantly slash one's risk for developing type 2 diabetes—a disease that has reached epidemic levels in North America. Researchers surmise that the DASH Diet can help improve blood sugar levels.
- Data is clear that switching from a Western-style diet replete with processed foods to one rich in whole foods as dictated by the DASH Diet can help people trim their waistline.
- An *American Journal of Epidemiology* study concluded that a diet high in fruits and vegetables, such as the DASH Diet, was associated with a lower risk of breast cancer.
- Eating more whole foods may help you build bones of steel. Scientists at Duke University Medical Center found that the DASH Diet paired with reduced sodium intake can have beneficial effects on bone health by reducing bone turnover.
- Another Duke University Medical Center study suggests that pairing exercise with the DASH Diet can improve brain function such as memory and learning.
- A recent report in the *Journal of Nutrition* reported that subjects who followed a DASH Diet rich in fruits, vegetables, whole grains, and low-fat dairy products while low in saturated fat, total fat, cholesterol, refined grains, and sweets, with a total sodium intake of 2400 milligrams per day for 2 months witnessed drops in markers

of heart-hampering inflammation and levels of fibrinogen, a protein that contributes to blood clotting, which can raise the risk for suffering a heart attack.

- One study found that a DASH-style diet can be protective against kidney stone formation, while another report demonstrates it may be effective at improving mood.

- A 2011 investigation in the journal *Diabetes Care* showed that subjects adhering to the DASH Diet for eight weeks experienced a rise in their HDL "good" cholesterol numbers and a drop in their LDL "bad" cholesterol, making this diet a champion for heart health. In fact, scientists at the Johns Hopkins University School of Medicine suggest that the DASH Diet can reduce one's risk of developing heart disease in the next ten years by up to 18 percent.

Sodium Shakedown

While just 500 milligrams a day is necessary for good health, the most recent data from the CDC suggests the average American is feasting on 3,300 milligrams of sodium daily. Current dietary guidelines recommend curtailing daily intake at 2,300 milligrams or 1,500 milligrams or less for certain populations such as those with hypertension or diabetes.

For certain people, an excess of sodium can raise blood pressure, and, in turn, heighten the risk for heart disease, stroke, and kidney disease. For this reason, the DASH Diet preaches the importance of limiting your intake. A 2012 report in the *American Journal of Medicine* stated that salt intake reduction among the general population can represent a simple cost-saving way to reduce cardiovascular morbidity and mortality. Here are some ways to shake the salt habit:

- Compare labels when purchasing items such as condiments, frozen foods, cereals, and breads in the pursuit of the lowest sodium options.

- The majority of Americans' sodium intake comes from restaurant meals and fast-food. Use this cookbook to prepare more of your own meals, which gives you control of the salt shaker.

- Watch out for low-fat products. Many manufactures make up for the flavor lost when fat is removed from packaged items by dousing them with more salt.

- Go back to nature. If your meals come from a box or can, you probably eat too much sodium. Switch to a diet based on whole foods, which are naturally low in sodium—even when you salt them to taste.
- Spice is nice: Spices like cumin, cayenne, and curry can make food explode with flavor, allowing you to cut back on the amount of salt that is needed. Plus, they're excellent sources of disease-thwarting antioxidants.

Getting Started

The chart below is designed to make it easier to know how much of each food group to eat daily. It gives options for 1,200- and 2,000-calorie diets, but you may need to adjust the number of servings in each category based on your own caloric needs. A dietician can help determine more exactly what's right for you.

DASH Servings per Day		
Food Groups	1,200 calories per day	2,000 calories per day
Grains	3	4–5
Vegetables	4–5	5–6
Fruits	4	5–6
Low-fat and nonfat dairy	2–3	3
Lean meats, poultry, and fish	3–6 oz	6–7 oz
Nuts, seeds, and legumes	3–4 per week	4–5 per week
Fats and oils	2	3
Sweets and added sugars	0	fewer than 5 per week

According to the National Institutes of Health, to be DASH compliant, a serving of grains is a slice of bread, or about ½ cup cooked rice, pasta, or cereal. One serving of dairy equals 1 cup milk or yogurt, or 1½ ounces cheese. One ounce of cooked meat, poultry, or fish is one serving, as is one whole egg. A serving of nuts, seeds, and legumes is ⅓ cup or 1½ ounces nuts, 2 tablespoons peanut butter or seeds, or ½ cup cooked legumes like beans and peas. Fats and oils should be limited to 1 teaspoon butter or oil, 1 tablespoon mayonnaise, or 2 tablespoons salad dressing. One serving of sweets and sugars is 1 tablespoon sugar, jelly, or jam and ½ cup sorbet.

If you've eaten a certain way for a number of years, you may initially find the DASH Diet a challenge to implement. Here are some tips to make the transition less arduous:

- Start by replacing one refined grain with a whole grain option each week. So you could choose 100-percent whole wheat bread for your lunch sandwich instead of bread made with white flour or swap out white rice for brown rice.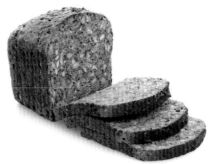
- Sneak fruits into more meals and snacks. Try adding extra berries to your morning cereal, toss some orange segments onto a dinner salad, or pack an apple with your lunch.
- Use frozen vegetables and pre-sliced fresh versions to make adding veggies into your diet more convenient.
- Try shopping more often at farmers' markets, which can supply a bounty of DASH-approved foods like local vegetables at very reasonable prices.
- Gradually cut back on the amount of salt you add to your meals. So, if you are used to adding ½ teaspoon salt to soups, lower this amount to ¼ teaspoon. Studies suggest your taste buds will adjust and soon you'll appreciate lower-sodium foods. Also, remove the salt shaker from the dining table.
- Commit to trying one recipe from this cookbook per week.
- Once a week, swap out red meat for other lean protein choices like chicken breast, salmon, or beans.
- Consider getting friends, family members, and office mates on board with the DASH Diet and take up the challenge together. The encouragement of others can really help make success more likely.

On the Move

No healthy eating plan such as the DASH Diet should be undertaken without the inclusion of physical activity. Case in point: A study in the prestigious *Archives of Internal Medicine* reported that the addition of exercise to the DASH Diet resulted in even greater reductions in blood pressure in subjects. University of Rhode Island researchers determined that the addition of resistance training to dietary education centered around the DASH Diet was more effective at slashing cardiovascular-disease risk factors than when subjects only received dietary counseling. Furthermore, a study in the journal *Hypertension* concluded that overweight subjects who followed the DASH Diet and incorporated regular exercise into their lifestyle improved their insulin sensitivity (which slashes diabetes risk) and blood fat levels (offering protection from heart disease) to a much greater degree than those who dieted without any physical activity.

Sadly, about seven out of ten American adults don't exercise regularly despite the proven health benefits. But you don't have to scale a mountain or lift iron in the gym for two hours a day to reap the benefits of exercise.

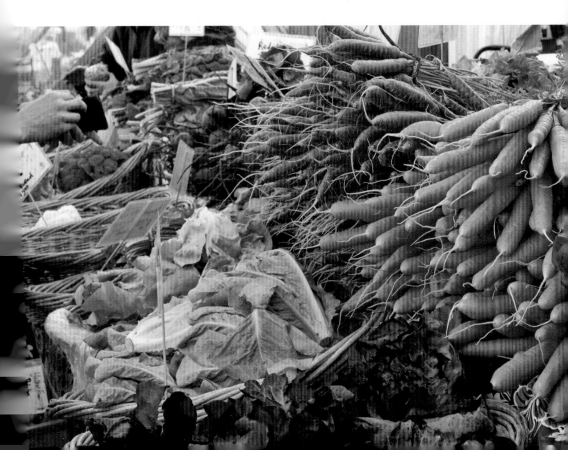

Start by incorporating thirty minutes of activity such as walking or swimming into your daily routine and build up from there. And don't overlook the importance of resistance training. Lifting weights builds lean body mass, which boosts fat-burning metabolism. Losing body fat is a proven way to lower blood pressure numbers and keep your heart beating strong.

APPETIZERS AND SNACKS

Think you need to make appetizers or snacks just for special occasions? Think again. Not only are they a fun and flavorful way to start a meal, but they also make great snacks throughout the day, or have a few for a light lunch. For example, cherry tomatoes dipped in hummus are a common afternoon snack at my home, and spring rolls are often a lunch indulgence.

Of course, it's helpful to have a few appetizer recipes in your repertoire to serve when company comes. A flavorful appetizer doesn't have to be complicated. Often, a good recipe merely combines a few complementary ingredients, transforming them into magic. And while many appetizers can be overly generous in calories, fat, and sodium, as these recipes demonstrate, it's entirely possible to create DASH-friendly dishes that require minimal prep work yet have plenty of spark to wake up your taste buds.

Spring Rolls

With scallions, basil, and hoisin, you can pack a lot of flavor into a small spring roll wrapper. The soft, creamy avocado provides a great contrast to the crunch of the carrots and radishes. You can find hoisin sauce and spring roll wrappers in the Asian section of most grocers. MAKES 10 TO 12 SPRING ROLLS

½ English cucumber, peeled

1 medium carrot

6 radishes

2 scallions, chopped

1 (10.5-ounce) package spring roll wrappers

2 tablespoons hoisin sauce, plus more to serve

12 basil leaves

1 avocado, sliced (see page 137)

Position a box grater in a medium bowl. Grate the cucumber, carrot, and radishes into the bowl, and add the scallions. Stir together the vegetables, then blot with paper towels to absorb excess moisture. Fill another medium bowl with cold water. Individually soak each spring roll wrapper in the cold water for 15 to 30 seconds until pliable. Place the wrapper on a flat work surface. Spread ½ teaspoon hoisin sauce in a line down the center of the wrapper. Fill with 1 basil leaf, 1 slice of avocado, and 1½ tablespoons filling. Roll the wrapper over the mixture once, then fold in the sides and roll to close. Repeat for the remaining wrappers. Serve with additional hoisin sauce.

DO THE DASH   The DASH diet encourages eating plenty of nutrient-plush vegetables, so look for ways to incorporate them into more recipes such as this appetizer. Though high in fat, avocados are not to be feared. The fat they contain is mostly monounsaturated, which has been shown to help improve cholesterol levels.

SHOPPING TIP   If a few different bottles of hoisin sauce are available at your grocery store, compare the sodium levels and select the one with the least amount. Made from soybean paste, it's considered by some chefs to be the equivalent of Chinese barbecue sauce.

NUTRITION   Per Spring Roll: 130 calories; 4 grams protein; 22 grams carbohydrate; 2 grams fiber; 3 grams fat (0.5 gram saturated); 232 mg sodium

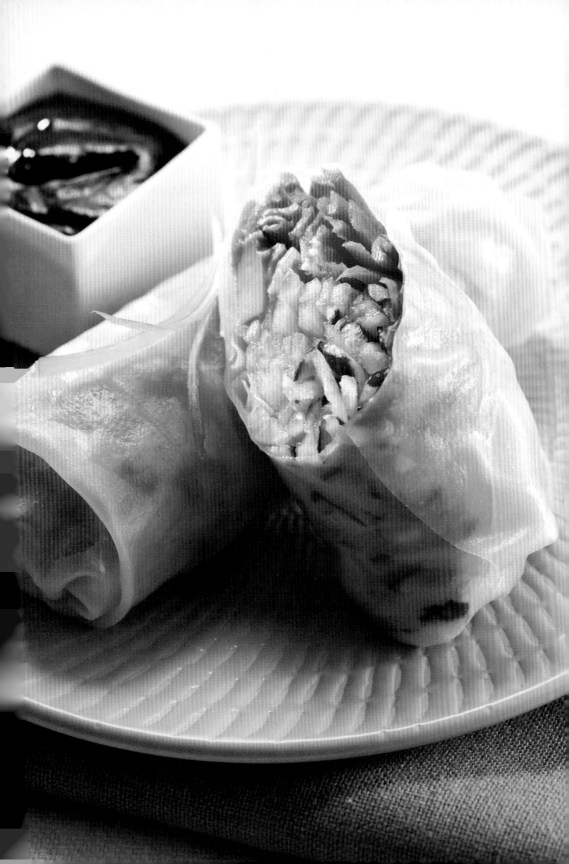

Arugula and Salami—Stuffed Peppadew Peppers

Peppadew peppers are a sweet pepper soaked in a pickling brine, giving them a sweet-and-sour appeal. You can find them at the deli counter or olive bar at most grocers. You can rinse them if you want to remove any excess sodium. *MAKES 10 PEPPERS*

10 Peppadew peppers, drained

3 to 4 tablespoons low-fat cream cheese (neuchâtel)

1 teaspoon canola oil

3 tablespoons chopped salami

1 (5-ounce) package arugula

Arrange the peppers on a plate. Fill each pepper with about 1 teaspoon cream cheese. Heat the canola oil in a medium nonstick sauté pan or skillet over medium-high heat. Add the salami and cook, stirring constantly, 1 to 2 minutes. Add the arugula and cook, stirring constantly, until wilted, 2 to 4 minutes. Remove from the heat. Fill each pepper with an equal portion of the salami arugula mixture. Serve.

DO THE DASH   Here's a great example of where the vegetables are the star of the show, with meat and cheese playing only a supporting roll. Try this concept more often for meals as well to reach the DASH-recommended 4 to 6 servings of veggies a day.

SHOPPING TIP   It's worth paying a visit to a well-stocked deli counter, which may offer cured meats like salami that are lower in sodium than packaged deli meats and free of potentially harmful preservatives like nitrates.

NUTRITION   Per Serving: 143 calories; 7 grams protein; 5 grams carbohydrate; 1 gram fiber; 11 grams fat (4 grams saturated); 461 mg sodium

Roasted Tomato Bruschetta

This version of bruschetta, an antipasto hailing from Italy, is loaded with tomato-garlic goodness and is sure to disappear from the appetizer platter quickly. If time is a concern, you can use store-bought packaged crostini, but try to find a whole-grain option.   *SERVES 4*

1 loaf whole wheat French bread, thinly sliced

2 pints cherry tomatoes, halved

4 cloves garlic, peeled

1 tablespoon extra-virgin olive oil

¼ teaspoon kosher salt

¼ teaspoon freshly ground black pepper

2 tablespoons chopped basil

Preheat the oven to 375°F. Spread the bread slices on a baking sheet, lightly brush the tops with olive oil, and bake until toasted, about 10 minutes. Remove the bread slices from the oven and raise the temperature to 425°F. Line a rimmed baking sheet with foil. Spread the tomatoes and the garlic on the prepared baking sheet. Drizzle with the olive oil and sprinkle with the salt and pepper. Toss to coat with the olive oil and seasonings. Roast until the tomatoes are crinkly and collapsed, 30 to 35 minutes, turning the baking sheet once halfway through cooking. Set aside to cool. Use your hands to combine the tomatoes and the garlic. Taste the spread and adjust the seasoning, if needed. To serve, spread the tomato mixture onto each crostini and garnish with the basil.

DO THE DASH   The DASH diet is big on eating the rainbow for a greater variety of heart-healthy nutrients and antioxidants. The red in cherry tomatoes comes from the antioxidant lycopene which may help reduce cardiovascular disease risk.

SHOPPING TIP   When purchasing bread products, make sure the first ingredient listed is a whole grain such as whole wheat or whole rye. Some bread labeled "made with whole grain," is still predominantly white flour.

NUTRITION   Per Serving: 201 calories; 9 grams protein; 30 grams carbohydrate; 6 grams fiber; 6 grams fat (1 gram saturated); 441 mg sodium

Shrimp with Spicy Cocktail Sauce

Cocktail sauce is a snap to make and provides a wallop of taste that's not apparent with the jarred variety. Plus, making your own helps to cut down on sodium levels. *SERVES 4*

1 cup ketchup, preferably low-salt

1½ tablespoons prepared horseradish

1 teaspoon grated lemon zest

1 tablespoon freshly squeezed lemon juice

2 teaspoons hot sauce, like Sriracha

1 pound frozen peeled, cooked shrimp, thawed

Combine the ketchup, horseradish, lemon zest, lemon juice, and hot sauce in a medium bowl. Taste the sauce and adjust the ingredients, as needed. Serve with the cold cooked shrimp.

DO THE DASH When choosing proteins, the DASH diet encourages lean choices. With just 85 calories and no saturated fat in a 3-ounce serving, shrimp is always a good candidate.

SHOPPING TIP Some brands like Heinz are now offering low-salt or salt-free ketchup options, which make this appetizer even more guilt-free.

NUTRITION Per Serving: 175 calories; 25 grams protein; 17 grams carbohydrate; 0 grams fiber; 1 gram fat (0 gram saturated); 340 mg sodium

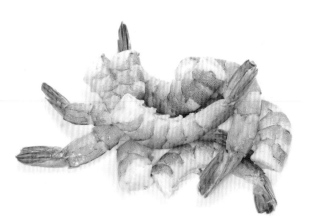

Black-Eyed Pea Dip

Black-eyed peas bring good luck on New Year's, but this dip can be enjoyed any time of year. The roasted tomatoes add a lot of flavor depth. Scoop up with tortilla chips. *SERVES 4*

1 pint grape tomatoes, halved
½ small red onion, coarsely chopped
1 tablespoon extra-virgin olive oil
1 jalapeño chile, seeded and chopped
1 roasted red bell pepper, chopped
1 (15-ounce) can black-eyed peas, rinsed and drained

1 tablespoon freshly squeezed lemon juice
1 tablespoon chopped cilantro
¼ teaspoon kosher salt
¼ teaspoon freshly ground black pepper
Multi-grain tortilla chips

Preheat the broiler. Line a rimmed baking sheet with foil, and add the tomatoes and onion. Drizzle the olive oil over top the vegetables, tossing to coat. Broil until semi-charred, 4 to 5 minutes, watching closely to prevent burning. Meanwhile, combine the jalapeño, bell pepper, black-eyed peas, lemon juice, cilantro, salt, and pepper in a medium bowl. Add the tomatoes and onions to the bowl and stir to combine. Serve with chips.

DO THE DASH The DASH Diet recommends 3 to 6 servings of fiber and nutrient-packed legumes a week. However, most Americans barely consume any legumes such as lentils and black-eyed peas. To ramp up your intake, incorporate them into dips, salads, and soups more often.

SHOPPING TIP When selecting chips for parties or the big game, opt for those that are baked and beefed up with healthier whole-food ingredients like flax, quinoa, blue corn, sweet potato, and even black beans.

NUTRITION Per Serving (without chips): 187 calories; 8 grams protein; 31 grams carbohydrate; 9 grams fiber; 4 grams fat (1 gram saturated); 405 mg sodium

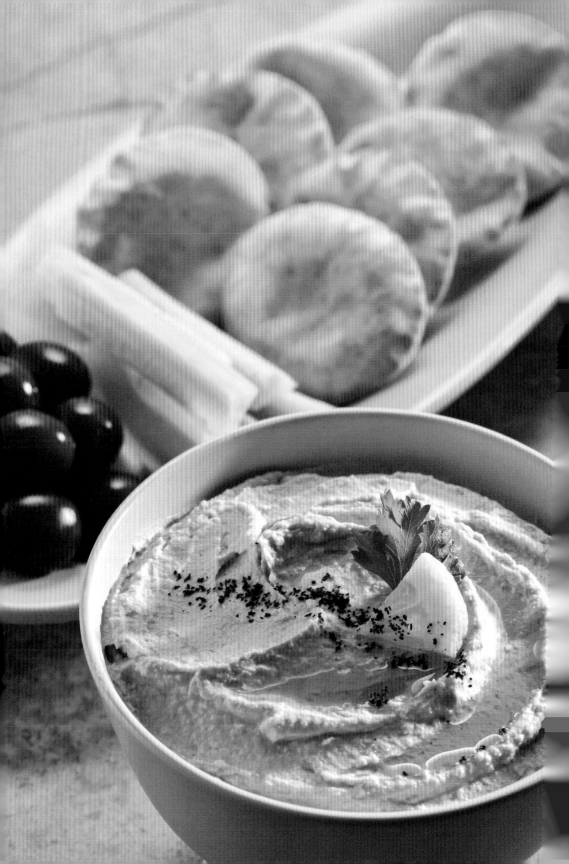

Hummus with Cucumber Slices and Cherry Tomatoes

For this hummus recipe, the traditional component tahini is left out. It's not a mistake—tahini (sesame paste) is a little expensive, and when I buy it, it usually lingers in the fridge because not many other recipes call for tahini. The slightly nontraditional hummus still shines without it. Serve with whole grain pita wedges and/or vegetable slices. *SERVES 4*

2 cloves garlic

1 (15-ounce) can chickpeas, rinsed and drained, 1 tablespoon liquid reserved

Grated zest and juice of 1 lemon

1 teaspoon sweet paprika

¼ teaspoon kosher salt

¼ teaspoon freshly ground black pepper

¼ cup extra-virgin olive oil, more or less

Fresh parsley, for garnish (optional)

2 cucumbers, sliced, to serve (optional)

1 pint cherry tomatoes, to serve

2 whole-grain pita breads, quartered, to serve (optional)

In a food processor, puree the garlic, chickpeas, reserved chickpea liquid, lemon zest, lemon juice, paprika, salt, and pepper. With the food processor running, pour in the olive oil through the feed tube and process until emulsified. Taste the hummus, and adjust the salt and lemon juice, if needed. Top with an extra drizzle of olive oil, a sprinkle of paprika, and parsley, if using. Serve with cucumber slices, tomatoes, and pita, if desired.

DO THE DASH Legumes such as chickpeas are brimming with fiber. By helping to keep you feeling full, fiber can aid in shedding pounds by reducing overeating. Giving canned beans a good rinse can greatly reduce their sodium levels.

SHOPPING TIP A few brands such as Eden are now offering beans that come in cans free of bisphenol-A (BPA). Some studies suggest that high blood levels of the sketchy chemical BPA can raise heart disease risk.

NUTRITION Per Serving: 249 calories; 5 grams protein; 25 grams carbohydrate; 5 grams fiber; 15 grams fat (2 grams saturated); 360 mg sodium

Guacamole with Pomegranate Seeds

Homemade guacamole is so easy to make, and much tastier than the store-bought kind. Conveniently, you can find pomegranate seeds in the produce section of most supermarkets. *SERVES 4*

2 ripe avocados, diced

2 tablespoons chopped cilantro

1 scallion, finely chopped

Juice of ½ lime

¼ teaspoon kosher salt

¼ cup pomegranate seeds

Multigrain tortilla chips, to serve

In a small bowl, mash the avocado using a fork. Add the cilantro, scallion, lime juice, salt, and half the pomegranate seeds and mix. Garnish with the remaining pomegranate seeds, and serve with tortilla chips.

DO THE DASH Not only do pomegranate seeds add a sweet-tart crunch to this guac, they are brimming with disease-thwarting antioxidants. Also, they team up with avocado to make this dip a fiber powerhouse.

SHOPPING TIP If your grocer only has rock-hard avocados but company is coming soon, you can hasten the ripening process by placing them in a brown paper bag and storing at room temperature. Adding an apple, tomato, or banana to the bag will speed up the ripening process by producing more ethylene gas.

NUTRITION Per Serving (without tortilla chips): 173 calories; 2 grams protein; 11 grams carbohydrate; 7 grams fiber; 15 grams fat (2 grams saturated); 154 mg sodium

Caramelized Onion Dip

I love caramelized onions as the caramelization process brings out their natural sweetness. But be patient—don't brown the onions too quickly—and you'll be justly rewarded. *SERVES 4*

1½ tablespoons canola oil

4 cups chopped yellow onions

¼ teaspoon kosher salt

2½ tablespoons low-fat mayonnaise

3 tablespoons crème fraîche

2 teaspoons freshly squeezed lemon juice

Whole-grain chips or crackers, to serve

Heat the canola oil in a large sauté pan or skillet over medium-high heat. Add the onions and salt, coating in the oil. Decrease the heat to medium-low, and cook the onions, stirring every couple of minutes. Monitor the onions to ensure they caramelize but do not burn. If the onions are cooking too quickly, decrease the heat. Let the onions cook about 25 minutes. Remove from heat and stir in the mayo, crème fraîche, and lemon juice. Taste the dip and adjust the ingredients as needed. Transfer to a bowl, cover, and refrigerate for several hours. Serve with chips or crackers.

DO THE DASH Dips are notoriously calorie bombs. Make them less hazardous to your waistline by using lower-fat versions of cheese and mayonnaise when possible and making sure you don't dunk too often. You can also try thick, protein-packed Greek-style yogurt as a replacement for mayonnaise, sour cream, and crème fraîche.

SHOPPING TIP With a high smoke point, canola oil is a top-notch cooking oil, but most of what is on the market is made from genetically modified rapeseed plants. If you prefer to avoid genetically modified products, you can do so by selecting organic-certified canola oil.

NUTRITION Per Serving (without chips or crackers): 169 calories; 2 grams protein; 15 grams carbohydrate; 2 grams fiber; 15 grams fat (2 grams saturated); 222 mg sodium

Cheese Log with Apple Slices

Cheddar cheese and apple is a classic flavor pairing. Spreading this cheese log onto apple slices is a nice way to contrast the creaminess of the softened cheese with the crisp bite of apple. *SERVES 4*

4 ounces reduced-fat sharp cheddar cheese, coarsely chopped

1½ ounces reduced fat cream cheese (neufchatel)

1 scallion, coarsely chopped

2 teaspoons Worcestershire sauce

½ cup unsalted walnuts, chopped, divided

Sliced apples such as Granny Smith, Gala, or Red Delicious, as needed

Add the cheddar cheese, cream cheese, scallion, Worcestershire sauce, and ¼ cup of the walnuts to a food processor. Pulse until smooth, about 1 to 2 minutes, stopping once to scrape down the mixture. Transfer the cheese mixture to waxed paper, and mold into a log shape. Sprinkle on the remaining ¼ cup walnuts. Wrap the entire log in waxed paper, and refrigerate for a few hours. Serve with apple slices.

DO THE DASH   The DASH diet suggests 2 to 4 servings of low-fat dairy each day as some data suggests that it can help control blood pressure numbers. Experiment with different reduced-fat cheese brands to find one that pleases your palate the most.

SHOPPING TIP   The bulk bins are a great place to find an assortment of heart-healthy nuts like omega-3–rich walnuts but make sure to choose only those that are labeled "unsalted." It's also wise to compare sodium levels on cheese as they can vary widely.

NUTRITION   Per Serving (without apples): 169 calories; 10 grams protein; 4 grams carbohydrate; 1 gram fiber; 13 grams fat (3 grams saturated); 249 mg sodium

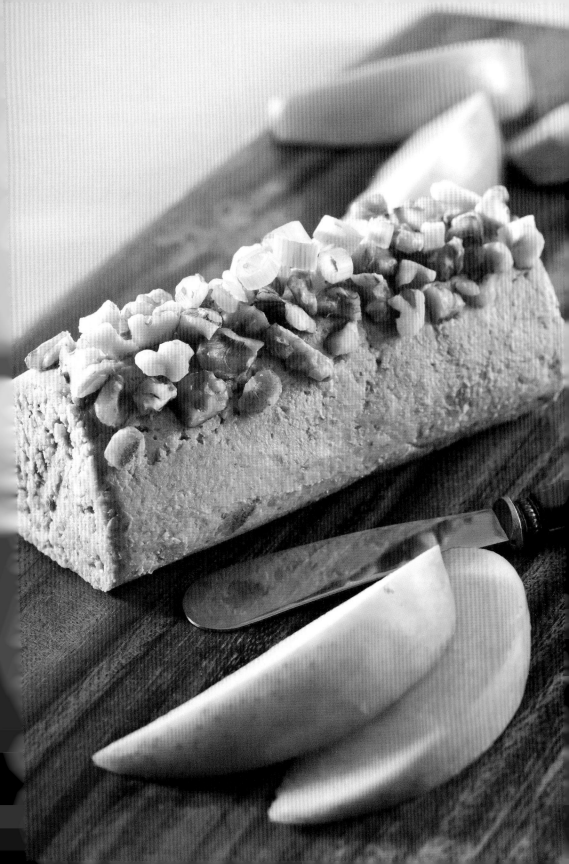

SALADS AND SOUPS

Canned soups are so convenient that too many people have forgotten how delicious a bowl of homemade soup can be. Simmering a pot of soup on the stove allows all the fresh flavors to meld in a way that simply can't come from a can. Soup brings back comforting memories of childhood and can be an easy way to explore new cuisines. Another reason soup is a pleasure to make is the ease of cooking it—you don't have to worry much about overcooking or undercooking. Plus, making your own lets you cut down on much of the sodium that is pumped into most canned versions, making them much more DASH Diet friendly.

Salads are another menu item that it's easy to get lazy about. Sure, you can fill your vegetable quota by grabbing a bag of premixed salad greens and dumping bottled dressing on top. But if you spend a little extra time mixing fresh ingredients, you will be rewarded with some really delicious results. It's easy to fall into a salad rut, so the recipes in this chapter add a little variety that will banish the humdrum from your salads.

Panzanella Salad

One of my favorite salads, panzanella is a salad hailing from Italy that is centered on tomatoes, olives, and bread cubes soaked in salad dressing. If you're not the kind of person who likes to sop up leftover sauce with bread, try substituting mini mozzarella balls (ciliegine) for the bread cubes. *Serves 4*

1 teaspoon Dijon mustard

¼ teaspoon kosher salt

1 tablespoon red wine vinegar

2½ tablespoons extra-virgin olive oil

2 cucumbers, peeled and cut into bite-size pieces

5 Roma tomatoes, cut into bite-size pieces

¼ cup pitted kalamata olives or other olive of your choice, coarsely chopped

1 large handful basil leaves (about 25 to 30 leaves)

2 cups bite-size cubes day-old firm bread, like French or Italian bread

Make the salad dressing: Whisk the mustard, salt, and vinegar in a small bowl to combine. Drizzle in the olive oil, whisking to emulsify. Taste and adjust the salt, vinegar, and olive oil, as needed.

In a large bowl, combine the cucumbers, tomatoes, olives, and basil. Pour half the salad dressing into the bowl, and toss with the salad mixture. Top the salad with the bread cubes and pour the remaining salad dressing over the bread. Let the salad sit for 15 to 20 minutes before serving so the bread cubes have time to absorb the dressing. Toss the salad to distribute the bread cubes, and serve.

DO THE DASH Tomatoes are a great way to add vitamin C to your diet. Researchers at Johns Hopkins University recently determined that higher intakes of vitamin C can reduce both systolic and diastolic blood pressure. Rinsing the olives can help remove some of the sodium from the brining liquid.

SHOPPING TIP Often, grocery stores mark down the price of day-old bread. So when shopping for the ingredients for this recipe, don't forget to look in the discount rack by the bread section.

NUTRITION Per Serving: 296 calories; 2 grams protein; 42 grams carbohydrate; 4 grams fiber; 11 grams fat (2 grams saturated); 640 mg sodium

Corn Salad

Fresh corn is a thing of beauty, but getting those kernels off the cob isn't. One of my favorite kitchen tools for the summer is OXO's Corn Stripper, and I swear they don't pay me to endorse it. What normally takes me 15 minutes to accomplish is done in just a few seconds with the Corn Stripper. Roasted red bell peppers can be found either in the olive bar or in the prepared foods aisle. *SERVES 4*

6 ears corn, shucked

¼ cup coarsely chopped cilantro

¼ cup finely chopped red onion

1 pint grape tomatoes, cut in half

2 roasted red bell peppers, diced (about 1 cup)

¼ teaspoon kosher salt

¼ teaspoon freshly ground black pepper

Juice of 1 lime

1½ tablespoons extra-virgin olive oil

In a large pot of boiling water, cook the ears of corn until the kernels have turned bright yellow, 3 to 4 minutes. Drain and let cool. When cool enough to handle, remove the corn kernels from the cob using a knife. Put the corn in a large bowl, and add the cilantro, red onion, tomatoes, bell peppers, salt, black pepper, lime juice, and olive oil. Toss the salad, taste, and adjust the seasonings as needed. Serve.

DO THE DASH The DASH diet preaches the importance of eating many different colors in order to consume as many different nutrients and antioxidants as possible. Here, we have yellow, green, and red.

SHOPPING TIP To save some money, you can try roasting your own red bell peppers. Simply place a whole pepper on the grill over medium heat and cook until slightly charred, turning every couple minutes.

NUTRITION Per Serving: 243 calories; 6 grams protein; 43 grams carbohydrate; 6 grams fiber; 7 grams fat (1 gram saturated); 152 mg sodium

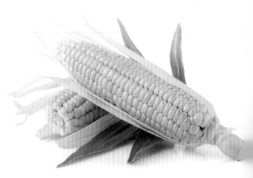

Spring Greens Salad with Fennel and Avocado

This is a nice basic salad with a simple homemade dressing and a sprinkle of sunflower seed kernels for added crunch. Salad dressing is so easy to make there's no reason to settle for store-bought. Plus, homemade often contains less sodium. *Serves 4*

1 teaspoon Dijon mustard

2 teaspoons honey

¼ teaspoon kosher salt

1½ tablespoons apple cider vinegar

¼ cup extra-virgin olive oil

1 (9-ounce) bag spring greens

4 Roma tomatoes, chopped

2 carrots, grated

2 medium fennel bulbs, trimmed of feathery stalks and thinly sliced

1 cucumber, peeled and chopped

1 ripe avocado, chopped (see page 137)

2 tablespoons unsalted sunflower seed kernels

Make the salad dressing: In a small bowl, whisk the mustard, honey, salt, and vinegar until combined. Drizzle in the olive oil, whisking to emulsify. Taste and adjust the salt, vinegar, and olive oil, as needed.

In a large bowl, add the greens, tomatoes, carrots, fennel, cucumber, and avocado. Lightly toss to combine. Drizzle with some of the dressing, toss, and taste, repeating until the ingredients are just coated. Sprinkle with the sunflower seed kernels and serve.

DO THE DASH Fennel has a pleasant licorice-like flavor plus good amounts of potassium, which is lauded in the DASH Diet as helping to keep blood pressure numbers in check. What's more, a 1-cup serving contains a mere 27 calories, making it waistline friendly.

SHOPPING TIP For ingredients not used so often, like sunflower seed kernels, it's cheaper and easier to nab just the amount you need from the bulk bins than to buy a large bag.

NUTRITION Per Serving: 298 calories; 5 grams protein; 22 grams carbohydrate; 9 grams fiber; 24 grams fat (4 grams saturated); 237 mg sodium

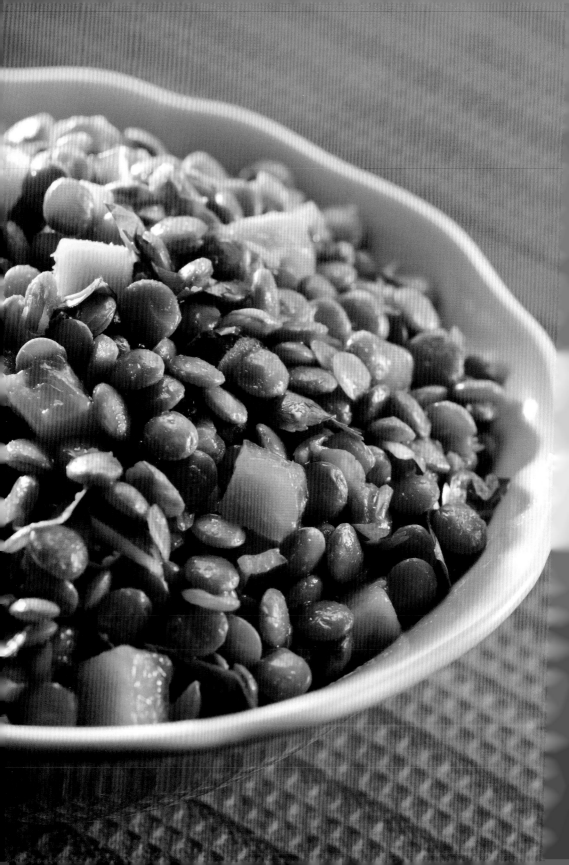

Lentil Salad with Mango

The bright flavors of mango, onion, and cilantro combine to make this an invigorating salad. *Serves 4*

1 cup dried green lentils

1 cup diced mango (about 1 large mango; see page 137)

1½ tablespoons chopped red onion

¼ cup chopped cilantro

½ tablespoon freshly squeezed lemon juice

1 tablespoon extra-virgin olive oil

In a medium saucepan, add the lentils and enough water to cover them by an inch or two. Bring to a boil, reduce the heat to low, and simmer, covered, until tender, about 20 minutes. Drain and let cool to room temperature.

In a medium bowl, add the lentils, mango, onion, and cilantro. Toss to combine. Drizzle with the lemon juice and the olive oil and toss again.

DO THE DASH   Inexpensive and versatile lentils are a great way to boost your intake of fiber (seriously, take a look at the fiber levels for this salad!). By helping keep blood sugar levels on an even keel, fiber can reduce hunger cravings and energy crashes.

SHOPPING TIP   By choosing dried lentils and beans more often, you'll not only lower your intake of sodium but also save a bit of cash. Dried lentils have the advantage of cooking much quicker than dried beans.

NUTRITION   Per Serving: 235 calories; 13 grams protein; 38 grams carbohydrate; 15 grams fiber; 4 grams fat (1 gram saturated); 5 mg sodium

Chinese Chicken Salad

With its large helping of chicken, this salad can serve as a healthy main course. The presence of orange in both the dressing and the salad nicely brings the whole dish together, which is also bolstered by the crunch of water chestnuts. *SERVES 4*

Juice of 2 oranges

2 tablespoons reduced-sodium soy sauce

2 teaspoons poppy seeds

1 tablespoon honey

2 tablespoons extra-virgin olive oil

½ medium head red cabbage, thinly sliced

1 head romaine lettuce, chopped

2 scallions, chopped

1 cucumber, peeled and chopped

1 avocado, diced

1 (8-ounce) can sliced water chestnuts, rinsed and drained

1 (11-ounce) can mandarin oranges, drained

3 cups shredded cooked chicken

Make the dressing: In a small bowl, whisk the orange juice, soy sauce, poppy seeds, and honey until combined. Continue whisking, slowly adding the olive oil, until emulsified. Reserve until needed.

Combine the cabbage and lettuce in a large bowl. Add the scallions, cucumber, avocado, water chestnuts, mandarin oranges, and chicken. Toss to combine. When ready to serve, toss with the dressing.

DO THE DASH   The average American only gets 2 to 3 servings of fruits and vegetables combined each day, so try making salads such as this on a Sunday afternoon and bring it to the office for healthy weekday lunches.

SHOPPING TIP   To cut down on prep work, you can use store-bought cooked rotisserie chicken for this salad. However, to keep fat calories down, make sure to discard the skin.

NUTRITION   Per Serving: 397 calories; 31 grams protein; 33 grams carbohydrate; 10 grams fiber; 19 grams fat (3 grams saturated); 603 mg sodium

Mixed Greens Soup

Just a little bacon is all that's needed to add oomph to this soup chock-full of healthy leafy green vegetables. To get a nice range of flavors, try to choose a variety of greens. SERVES 6

2 slices bacon, diced

1 medium onion, diced

2 cloves garlic, minced

3 cups chopped combined greens (spinach, collards, turnip greens, Swiss chard, or others)

4 cups low-sodium chicken broth

4 cups water

¼ teaspoon kosher salt

¼ teaspoon black pepper

In a large pot over medium-high heat, add the bacon, and stir until cooked but not crisp, 4 to 6 minutes. Add the onion and cook, stirring, until translucent, 2 to 3 minutes. Add the garlic and the greens, and cook briefly until the garlic is golden and the greens are wilted, 1 to 2 minutes. Add the chicken broth, water, salt, and pepper. Increase the heat to high, and bring the soup to a boil. Reduce the heat, and simmer until the flavors have melded, about 15 to 20 minutes.

Carefully transfer half of the soup to a food processor. Puree until smooth, about 1 minute. Return the pureed soup to the pot. Season to taste, and reheat the soup if necessary.

DO THE DASH   So jam-packed with essential nutrients, consider dark leafy greens like Swiss chard the MVPs of the produce department. Aim to consume at least 1 cup each day for good health.

SHOPPING TIP   Processed meats like bacon can blow the sodium budget; however, there are lower-sodium versions on the market, so compare the nutrition facts panel of several varieties. Many butchers can guide you toward their lowest-sodium options. There are now even no-salt-added chicken broths available.

NUTRITION   Per Serving: 41 calories; 4 grams protein; 4 grams carbohydrate; 1 gram fiber; 1 gram fat (0 grams saturated); 333 mg sodium

Chicken Soup with Crispy Rice

When I was a child, my mom learned how to make chicken soup with crispy fried rice. It was such a mess frying the rice in a vat of hot oil that we made it only once, but the sultry combination haunted me for years. Then I found frozen rice. The individual grains are frozen in a way that a quick stint in a sauté pan gives the same results I remember. *SERVES 4*

6 cups low-sodium chicken broth

¼ teaspoon salt

¼ teaspoon freshly ground black pepper

4 boneless, skinless chicken thighs

1 (20-ounce) package frozen brown rice

2 tablespoons canola oil

⅓ cup chopped scallions

In a medium pot over high heat, bring the chicken broth, salt, and pepper to a boil. Add the chicken thighs, cover, and reduce the heat to low. Simmer until the chicken is cooked through, 25 to 30 minutes. Cut into the thickest chicken piece to check that it's no longer pink. Take the pot off the heat, and transfer the chicken to a plate to cool. Shred the chicken with a fork, or cut into pieces. Return to the soup.

Heat the canola oil in a large nonstick skillet over high heat. Add one-half of the rice in one layer in the pan. Cook, undisturbed, until the rice is golden and crispy, 4 to 5 minutes. Transfer the rice to a plate. Add the remaining rice to the pan, and cook undisturbed for 3 to 4 minutes (the second batch will cook faster). To serve, ladle the chicken soup into bowls. Garnish with the crispy rice and the scallions.

DO THE DASH Many people are surprised to learn that dark poultry meat only contains an extra gram of saturated fat versus white meat per serving but actually have higher levels of certain minerals like iron and immune-boosting zinc. Plus, they tend to remain juicer during cooking and are often cheaper than white meat.

SHOPPING TIP Some manufactures pump their chicken full of a sodium rich broth, so make sure to read the fine print to assure the cuts you pick up have less than 100 milligrams per serving.

NUTRITION Per Serving: 286 calories; 18 grams protein; 29 grams carbohydrate; 2 grams fiber; 12 grams fat (2 grams saturated); 294 mg sodium

Potato Leek Soup

Creamy potato soup is always a treat, and is made even better by the addition of leeks. *SERVES 4*

1 tablespoon canola oil

3 medium leeks, sliced ¼ to ½ inch thick (see sidebar)

3 cups low sodium vegetable broth

1 pound red potatoes, diced

¼ teaspoon salt

¼ teaspoon black pepper

2 tablespoons crème fraîche

1 teaspoon dried dill, for garnish (optional)

Heat the canola oil in a medium pot over medium-high heat. Add the leeks and cook, stirring occasionally, until soft, about 10 minutes. Add the vegetable broth, potatoes, salt, and pepper, and bring to a boil. Lower the heat to medium-low and cook until the potatoes are tender and the soup is thickened, 25 to 30 minutes. Remove from the heat and, if you would like, use an immersion blender to puree the soup. You can also puree the soup in a blender or food processor and return to the pot. Season to taste, and stir in the crème fraîche. Ladle the soup into bowls and garnish with dill, if using.

DO THE DASH Though often wrongly maligned, potatoes are a rich source of potassium. Many studies suggest higher intakes of this electrolyte can help slash blood pressure numbers, perhaps by encouraging the kidney to excrete more sodium from the body.

SHOPPING TIP Substitute 2 percent Greek yogurt for the crème fraîche, it you want to lower the fat.

NUTRITION Per Serving: 190 calories; 3 grams protein; 30 grams carbohydrate; 3 grams fiber; 7 grams fat (2 grams saturated); 270 mg sodium

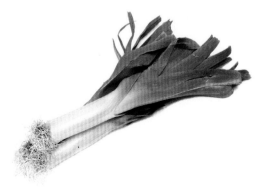

Turkey Chili with Beans

Chili always makes for a hearty, satisfying meal. When it's made with ground turkey and beans, it's a healthy complete meal in one pot. Serve the chili with your favorite garnishes, such as low-fat sour cream, shredded cheese, olives, diced avocado, or thinly sliced scallions. SERVES 6

2 teaspoons canola oil

1 pound lean ground turkey

2 yellow onions, finely chopped

2 red bell peppers, finely chopped

1 (28-ounce) can chopped tomatoes, including juice

1 (15½-ounce) can pinto beans, drained and rinsed

1 (15½-ounce) can black beans, drained and rinsed

¾ cup strongly brewed coffee

1 tablespoon chili powder, plus more as needed

3 cloves garlic, chopped

¼ teaspoon kosher salt

¼ teaspoon black pepper

Heat the canola oil in a Dutch oven over medium-high heat. Add the turkey and cook, stirring constantly to break up the meat into small pieces, until no longer pink, 6 to 8 minutes. Add the onion and the bell pepper, sautéing until soft, 5 to 7 minutes. Add the tomatoes, beans, and coffee, stirring to combine. Bring the mixture to a simmer, and add the chili powder, garlic, salt, and pepper. Lower the heat to medium-low, cover, and cook at a constant simmer until the flavors have melded, 30 to 45 minutes. Taste and adjust the seasonings, if needed. Ladle the chili into bowls and serve with garnishes.

DO THE DASH Chili is a great way to work more beans into your diet. As a leading source of dietary fiber, they can help boost satiety which helps reduce caloric intake and, in turn, unwelcome weight gain.

SHOPPING TIP Many times poultry is ground with the skin, which sends the fat levels soaring. Make sure you choose ground breast meat, which only contains the low-fat white meat. Also, look for lower-sodium canned beans.

NUTRITION Per Serving: 276 calories; 29 grams protein; 39 grams carbohydrate; 11 grams fiber; 2 grams fat (0 grams saturated); 632 mg sodium

SIDES

Sometimes, a great side dish makes the meal. Turkey is all right, but Thanksgiving is really all about the array of delicious sides like stuffing and sweet potatoes. Not every night can be as special as Thanksgiving, but serving a thoughtful, delicious side can make any meal more memorable. It's also a great way to work in additional DASH Diet–approved items such as vegetables and whole grains into a meal.

This chapter features new, healthier spins on comforting favorites, like mashed potatoes with the tang of buttermilk and creamed spinach with just a spoonful of crème fraîche to provide a hint of creaminess. There are also some dishes that will be less familiar, like cucumber briefly sautéed with pepper flakes or celery root and apple made into a puree. And why relegate side dishes to second-class status? Combine a few and feast to make a complete meal.

Pesto-Stuffed Tomatoes

As far as I'm concerned, you can never go wrong with pesto, Parmesan, or panko. I use all three together for these simple and sultry stuffed tomatoes. *SERVES 4*

2 tablespoons grated Parmigiano-Reggiano cheese

⅓ cup panko bread crumbs

1 tablespoon prepared pesto

4 small to medium tomatoes, hulled (see page 137)

Preheat the oven to 400°F. Combine the cheese and bread crumbs in a small bowl. Add the pesto, and stir to combine with the dry ingredients. Fill each tomato's cavity with the bread crumb mixture. Place the tomatoes in an ovenproof dish and bake until the tomatoes and the filling are hot and the tops are browned, about 15 minutes.

DO THE DASH   The DASH diet is high in antioxidant-rich foods such as tomatoes. In fact, tomato's signature cancer-fighting antioxidant lycopene is more available to the body when they are cooked.

SHOPPING TIP   Making your own pesto at home is far from difficult and lets you control the amount of salt added. Just search for pesto at www.foodgawker.com for plenty of inspiration.

NUTRITION   Per Serving: 84 calories; 3 grams protein; 11 grams carbohydrate; 2 grams fiber; 2 grams fat (1 gram saturated); 140 mg sodium

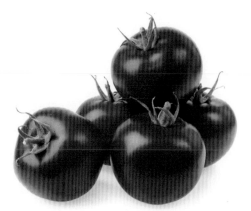

Polenta with Dried Mushrooms

While I chose the black trumpet mushrooms for this recipe, you can also use other varieties based on preference and cost. Because the dark mushroom stock is used to heighten the earthy flavor of the polenta, the shade is a bit murky—great to eat but not overly photo-worthy. *Serves 4*

½ ounce dried black trumpet mushrooms

1½ cups hot water

2 cups low-fat milk

½ teaspoon dried thyme

¼ teaspoon kosher salt

½ cup coarse cornmeal

1½ tablespoons unsalted butter

Soak the dried mushrooms in the water for 15 minutes. Drain the mushrooms through a fine-mesh sieve set over a 2-cup measure, and reserve the soaking liquid. Rinse the mushrooms, chop them, and reserve. Pour 1 cup of the soaking liquid into a medium pot, through the strainer again to make sure there's no dirt left. Add the milk, thyme, and salt, and bring to a boil over high heat. Add the cornmeal, whisking constantly. Turn down the heat, and let simmer until the polenta is as thick as you want it, 5 to 10 minutes. Stir in the butter. Taste and adjust the seasonings if necessary.

DO THE DASH Rehydrated dried mushrooms are a great way to add meaty texture to dishes for very few calories.

SHOPPING TIP Dried mushrooms can be expensive, but you'll often find the best deals in Asian markets.

NUTRITION Per Serving: 145 calories; 5 grams protein; 18 grams carbohydrate; 1 gram fiber; 6 grams fat (4 grams saturated); 205 mg sodium

Marinated Eggplant with Olives

This simple marinated eggplant recipe makes a nice Mediterranean-influenced warm-weather side. *SERVES 4*

3 medium Italian eggplants, sliced crosswise ½-inch thick

2 tablespoons extra-virgin olive oil

¼ teaspoon kosher salt

¼ teaspoon freshly ground black pepper

¼ cup chopped mint

⅓ cup pitted oil-cured black olives, coarsely chopped

Preheat the broiler. Line one or two rimmed baking sheets with foil, and add the eggplant. Drizzle with the olive oil and season with the salt and pepper. Broil the eggplant until slightly charred but still chewy, 3 to 4 minutes. Turn the eggplant over and broil 3 to 4 minutes longer. Remove from the broiler, and let cool. Repeat until all the eggplant has been broiled. When the eggplant has cooled, cut into bite-size pieces. Transfer to a bowl, and combine with the mint and the olives. Drizzle with additional olive oil. Serve the marinated eggplant cold or at room temperature.

DO THE DASH Because of the heightened flavor and texture nuisances of coarser salts such as kosher, Himalayan, and fleur de sel, you can often use much less on your food compared to typical table salt.

SHOPPING TIP It's cheaper to buy olives from the olive bar, so you can purchase just the amount you need and not a whole jar which might languish in the fridge. The quality and variety are better, too.

NUTRITION Per Serving: 142 calories; 3 grams protein; 17 grams carbohydrate; 10 grams fiber; 9 grams fat (1 gram saturated); 246 mg sodium

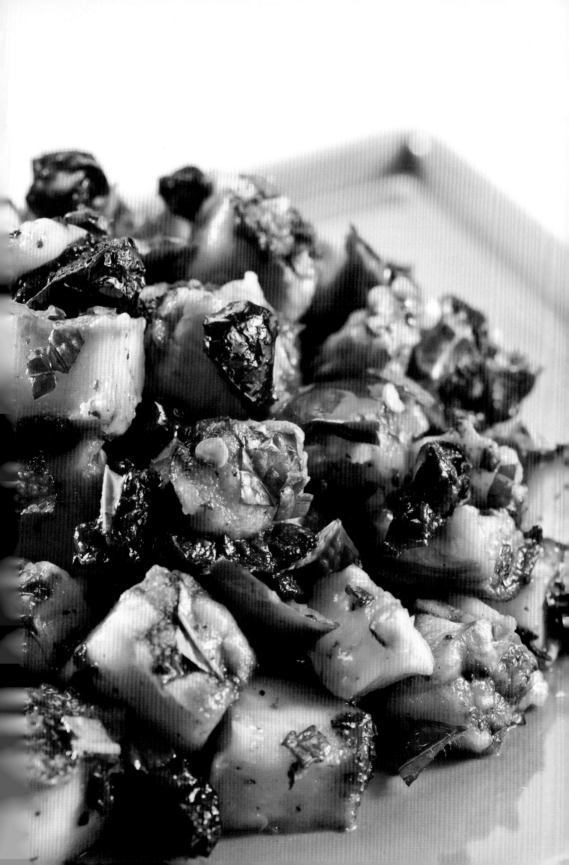

Low-Fat Creamed Spinach

Using reduced-fat versions of both cream cheese and Greek yogurt greatly reduces the fat in this recipe. The result isn't as creamy as full-fat creamed spinach, but it still tastes very rich and the yogurt gives it a pleasing tang. *SERVES 6*

2 (16-ounce) packages frozen chopped spinach, thawed

½ cup water

4 cloves garlic, minced

4 ounces reduced-fat cream cheese (neuchâtel)

½ cup low-fat milk

½ cup 2% Greek yogurt

¼ teaspoon salt

¼ teaspoon freshly ground black pepper

In a large pot over medium-high heat, cook the spinach in the water, stirring occasionally, until all the water evaporates, about 5 minutes. Stir in the garlic and cook 1 minute. Reduce the heat to low, add the cream cheese and the milk, stirring and cooking until the cream cheese is melted, 5 to 7 minutes. Remove from the heat and stir in the yogurt. Season with the salt and pepper, and serve.

DO THE DASH The recipe is a great way to get your necessary daily intake of leafy greens and low-fat dairy. Spinach is particularly abundant in vitamin K, which is needed to help build healthy bones.

SHOPPING TIP When possible, choose organic dairy products, which come from cows that are not administered hormones or antibiotics.

NUTRITION Per Serving: 107 calories; 10 grams protein; 10 grams carbohydrate; 4 grams fiber; 4 grams fat (2 grams saturated); 311 mg sodium

Celery Root and Apple Puree

Never used celery root before? Trust me, you're missing out. Celery root has a flavor that resembles celery and parsley and a texture that's similar to a potato or a parsnip. This dish is like mashed potatoes for those who think potatoes are a little bland. *Serves 4*

2 pounds celery root, peeled and cut into 1-inch pieces

2 red apples, peeled and sliced

2 tablespoons unsalted butter

½ cup low-fat milk

¼ teaspoon kosher salt

Add the celery root to a pot of salted water over high heat. When the water reaches a boil, add the apples and cook until the celery root is easily pierced with a knife, about 12 minutes. Reserving 1 cup of the cooking water, drain the celery root and apples and place in a food processor. Add the butter, milk, and salt. Puree until smooth, scraping down the sides if necessary. If you want a smoother consistency, add the reserved cooking water as needed. Serve at once.

DO THE DASH It might be the ugly duckling of the vegetable world, but celery root (aka celeriac) is a nutritional heavyweight with good amounts of vitamin C, fiber, blood pressure-lowering potassium, and vitamin K.

SHOPPING TIP When making dishes such as mashed potatoes or this version of a comfort food classic, try evaporated milk as a replacement for higher-fat half-and-half or heavy cream.

NUTRITION Per Serving: 207 calories; 5 grams protein; 35 grams carbohydrate; 6 grams fiber; 7 grams fat (4 grams saturated); 384 mg sodium

NOT ESPECIALLY FLAVORFUL. BUT A GOOD SNACK.

I like this — SS. Scott said it reminds him of baby food; that's pretty accurate. —an

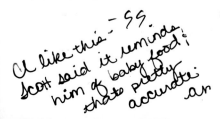

Roasted Brussels Sprouts with Mustard Seeds

Brussels sprouts sometimes get a bad rap, but they're one of my favorite vegetables. My preferred way to prepare Brussels sprouts is to roast them because the process heightens their natural sweetness. *SERVES 4*

1¼ pounds Brussels sprouts, ends trimmed and halved lengthwise

2½ tablespoons extra-virgin olive oil, divided

1 tablespoon freshly squeezed lemon juice

¼ teaspoon kosher salt

¼ teaspoon freshly ground black pepper

1½ teaspoons mustard seeds

Preheat the oven to 400°F. Line a rimmed baking sheet with foil. Spread the Brussels sprouts on the sheet and cover with 1½ tablespoons of the olive oil and the lemon juice, salt, and pepper. Toss to combine. Roast the sprouts until the outer leaves are crisped, about 45 minutes, rotating the baking sheet once midway through. Remove from the oven, and add the remaining 1 tablespoon olive oil and the mustard seeds. Toss to combine with the sprouts. Taste and adjust the seasonings as needed.

DO THE DASH Brussels sprouts have stellar amounts of vitamin C and vitamin K. Plus, a 1-cup serving only has 38 calories, so it should be part of a diet geared toward weight loss.

SHOPPING TIP Look for peppery whole mustard seeds in bulk bins or the spice aisle.

NUTRITION Per Serving: 154 calories; 6 grams protein; 16 grams carbohydrate; 7 grams fiber; 9 grams fat (1 gram saturated); 188 mg sodium

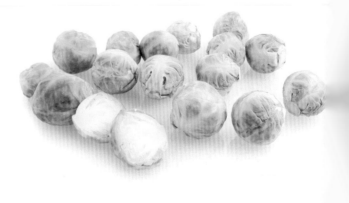

Quick-Sautéed Cucumbers with Red Pepper Flakes

I bet you never thought of cooking cucumbers, right? Neither did I, but one of my favorite Szechuan restaurants briefly sautés cucumbers over high heat to better infuse them with red pepper flakes. Just try it, and you'll be adding cooked cucumbers to your repertoire, too. *SERVES 4*

2 tablespoons extra-virgin olive oil

2 teaspoons dried red pepper flakes

2 cloves garlic, minced

1-inch piece fresh ginger, grated

3 English cucumbers, peeled, cut in half lengthwise, and cut into 1-inch pieces

1 tablespoon reduced-sodium soy sauce

Heat the olive oil in a large sauté pan or skillet over high heat. Add the pepper flakes, garlic, and ginger, and cook, stirring constantly, until fragrant, 15 to 30 seconds. Add the cucumber, stirring constantly to cook and combine with the other ingredients, about 1 minute. Add the soy sauce, and continue stirring for 1 more minute, scraping up any bits that have stuck to the bottom.

DO THE DASH The DASH diet recommends drinking plenty of water to stay well hydrated. One way to boost your intake of water is to eat plenty of low-calorie, water-rich fruits and vegetables such as cucumber.

SHOPPING TIP When shopping for Asian bottled items such as soy sauce, it's very important to compare the sodium levels of several options.

NUTRITION Per Serving: 82 calories; 1 gram protein; 4 grams carbohydrate; 1 gram fiber; 7 grams fat (1 gram saturated); 137 mg sodium

Buttermilk Mashed Potatoes

Substituting low-fat buttermilk for milk and cream cuts down on calories while adding a lovely tang to these mashed potatoes. *SERVES 4*

2 pounds russet potatoes (about 4 large)

½ teaspoon kosher salt

2 tablespoons unsalted butter

¾ cup low-fat buttermilk

2 tablespoons chopped chives, for garnish (optional)

Fill a large pot halfway with water. Chop the potatoes into medium pieces, as equal in size as possible. Add potatoes to pot and add more water if needed to cover. Bring to a boil over high heat. Cook until the potatoes are tender (stick a knife into a potato to check), 12 to 15 minutes. Drain the potatoes, and return to the pot. Add the salt, butter, and buttermilk. Use a potato masher to mash the potatoes until smooth, adding more buttermilk for the desired consistency, if needed. Taste and season with more salt, if needed, and garnish with chives, if using.

DO THE DASH Many recipes call for peeling the potatoes, but do so and you'll remove much of the nutritional value, including the dietary fiber that aids in weight loss, which helps with lowering blood pressure numbers. Adding more fresh herbs such as chives to dishes bolsters flavor without the need for more salt.

SHOPPING TIP Forgot to pick up buttermilk at the grocery store? You can essentially make your own by placing 1 tablespoon lemon juice in a 1-cup measuring cup and topping with regular milk. Stir and let sit for a few minutes.

NUTRITION Per Serving: 241 calories; 6 grams protein; 44 grams carbohydrate; 5 grams fiber; 6 grams fat (4 grams saturated); 353 mg sodium

Smashed "Fried" Potatoes

"Fried" is a misnomer here because the crispiness of the smashed potatoes comes from a stint in the oven, so this recipe is both easier to make and healthier to consume than one involving frying. Win, win. *SERVES 6*

8 medium red potatoes (about 1½ pounds)

2 tablespoons extra-virgin olive oil

½ teaspoon kosher salt

¼ teaspoon freshly ground black pepper

Add the potatoes to a large pot and fill three-quarters full with water, making sure to cover the potatoes. Bring to a boil over high heat and cook the potatoes until almost tender, about 30 minutes. Drain and let cool.

Preheat the oven to 450°F. Line a rimmed baking sheet with foil. When the potatoes are cool enough to handle, halve lengthwise. Place the potato halves cut-side up on the prepared baking sheet. Using a potato masher, gently press down on the potatoes to flatten. (You don't want to press so hard that the potatoes break into a many pieces. Just press gently to flatten them.) Season with the olive oil, salt, and pepper. Roast the potatoes until slightly browned and crispy on top, about 30 minutes.

DO THE DASH   On top of containing plenty of blood pressure–lowering potassium, researchers in the U.K. discovered spuds possess molecules called kukoamines, believed to also help lower blood pressure numbers. Remember, keep the skin on for added nutrition.

SHOPPING TIP   When purchasing black pepper, consider choosing whole peppercorns and grinding them as needed in a pepper mill for better flavor and a longer shelf life.

NUTRITION   Per Serving: 258 calories; 6 grams protein; 52 grams carbohydrate; 6 grams fiber; 5 grams fat (1 gram saturated); 211 mg sodium

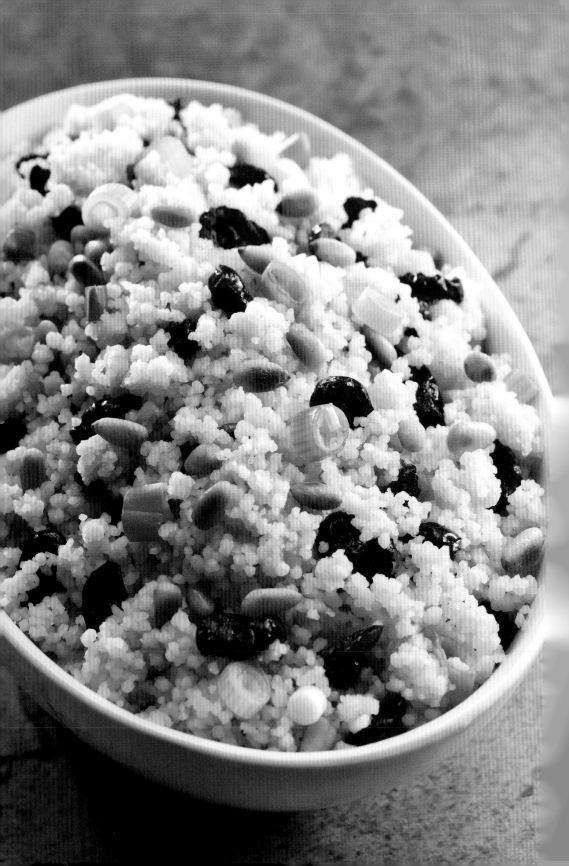

Couscous with Dried Cranberries and Pine Nuts

Couscous is a cinch to make but can be a little boring if you cook it in water. Using vegetable stock, or some other kind of broth, gives it a much richer flavor. The addition of pine nuts and cranberries makes this a well-rounded side that you'll be happy to eat on a regular basis.   *Serves 4*

2 teaspoons canola oil

¼ cup pine nuts

2 cups reduced-sodium vegetable stock

½ teaspoon kosher salt

¼ teaspoon freshly ground black pepper

1 cup couscous, preferably whole wheat

⅓ cup dried cranberries

2 scallions, coarsely chopped

Heat the canola oil in a medium pot over medium-high heat. Add the pine nuts, cooking until lightly browned, 2 to 3 minutes, stirring constantly. Add the vegetable stock, salt, and pepper. Bring to a boil and add the couscous and cranberries. Remove from the heat, cover with a lid, and let sit for 10 minutes. Fluff the couscous and stir in the scallions. Taste and adjust the seasoning as needed.

DO THE DASH   With the water removed, dried fruits like cranberries are a concentrated source of heart-healthy nutrients like antioxidants. However, they are higher in calories than their fresh counterparts, so portion control is prudent.

SHOPPING TIP   Once a rarity, most grocery stores are now carrying whole wheat couscous, which is a nutritional step up from its more refined counterpart.

NUTRITION   Per Serving: 283 calories; 7 grams protein; 45 grams carbohydrate; 3 grams fiber; 9 grams fat (1 gram saturated); 657 mg sodium

Kasha with Spring Vegetables

In late spring, you'll find fiddleheads, the furled fronds of a young fern, at farmers' markets and some grocery stores. Some stores now also sell them in their frozen vegetable section year round. Their flavor wanders somewhere between asparagus and broccoli. If you can't find them, try using asparagus with this recipe. Kasha is whole-grain roasted buckwheat, popular in Eastern Europe. It's a source of fiber, protein, magnesium, and manganese. *SERVES 4*

2 teaspoons extra-virgin olive oil

1 (9-ounce) bag fresh spinach

1 medium zucchini, grated

½ cup fiddleheads, or asparagus

2 cups reduced-sodium vegetable broth

1 cup kasha

¼ teaspoon kosher salt

¼ teaspoon freshly ground black pepper

Heat the olive oil in a medium pot over medium-high heat. Add the spinach, in batches if necessary, and stir until wilted. Add the zucchini and the fiddleheads, sautéing until softened and combined with the spinach, 2 to 3 minutes. Add the broth, kasha, salt, and pepper. Bring to a boil, cover, and reduce the heat to low. Simmer until the kasha is tender, about 15 minutes. Remove from the heat and fluff the kasha with a fork. Taste and adjust the seasoning as needed.

DO THE DASH   Fiddleheads contain a fantastic amount of nutrients including niacin, immune-boosting beta-carotene, vitamin C, and potassium, the latter two of which have been shown to help lower blood pressure numbers.

SHOPPING TIP   An excellent source for a range of DASH Diet–approved whole grains like kasha, quinoa, amaranth, and barley is www.bobsredmill .com.

NUTRITION   Per Serving: 204 calories; 8 grams protein; 38 grams carbohydrate; 6 grams fiber; 4 grams fat (1 gram saturated); 275 mg sodium

Curried Cauliflower with Dried Cherries

Cauliflower is an underrated vegetable. It has a subtle taste that allows it to pick up surrounding flavors such as curry powder. *SERVES 4*

1 tablespoon unsalted butter

2 teaspoons curry powder

½ teaspoon kosher salt

¼ teaspoon freshly ground black pepper

1 head cauliflower, cut into bite-size pieces

⅓ cup water

¼ cup dried cherries

Melt the butter in a large sauté pan or skillet over medium-high heat. Add the curry powder, salt, and pepper, and cook, stirring, until fragrant, 30 seconds. Add the cauliflower, and stir to combine with the butter and spices. Cook until slightly golden, 2 to 3 minutes. Add the water, and cover with a lid. Cook until the cauliflower is tender and the water has evaporated, 3 to 4 minutes longer. Stir in the cherries. Taste and adjust the seasonings as needed.

DO THE DASH The DASH diet is heavy on vegetables such as cauliflower, which is rich in vitamin C, vitamin K, and folate, a B vitamin shown to confer protection against certain cancers.

SHOPPING TIP If possible, look for dried cherries that are unsweetened to save on sugar calories. Like fresh, they are loaded with age-avenging antioxidants.

NUTRITION Per Serving: 84 calories; 3 grams protein; 14 grams carbohydrate; 4 grams fiber; 3 grams fat (2 grams saturated); 334 mg sodium

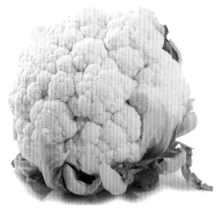

Roasted Asparagus with Orange Zest

I always look forward to asparagus season in the spring. Asparagus is often at its best when it's simply prepared, but I think it benefits from the addition of a little orange flavor. SERVES 4

2 bunches asparagus, trimmed (see page 138)

1½ tablespoons extra-virgin olive oil

Grated zest and juice of 1 orange

¼ teaspoon kosher salt

½ teaspoon freshly ground black pepper

Preheat the oven to 400°F. Line a rimmed baking sheet with foil, and spread the asparagus in rows. Drizzle with the olive oil and orange juice. Sprinkle with salt and pepper. Roast until the asparagus is tender, about 20 minutes. Garnish with the orange zest, and serve.

DO THE DASH   The DASH Diet stresses eating plenty of nutrient-dense foods. That is, foods that contain a large amount of nutrients in relation to their calories. At only 27 calories per 1-cup serving yet packed with folate, vitamin C, iron, and fiber, asparagus surely fits the bill.

SHOPPING TIP   When using citrus zest for recipes, you may want to splurge for organic since you are using the outside of the fruit that may contain pesticide residues.

NUTRITION   Per Serving: 99 calories; 5 grams protein; 11 grams carbohydrate; 5 grams fiber; 5 grams fat (1 gram saturated); 150 mg sodium

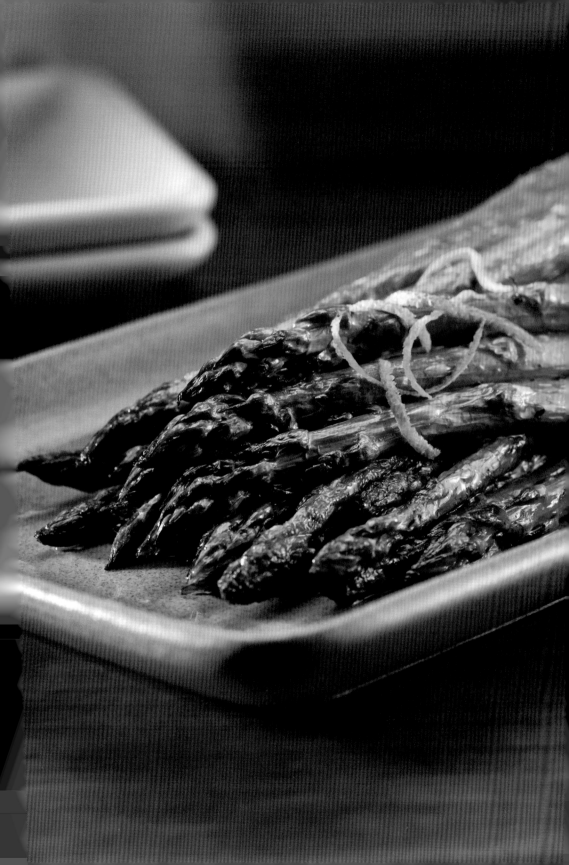

Braised Fennel with Oranges and Olives

The licorice-like flavor of fennel makes for an intriguing combination with briny olives and sweet oranges. *SERVES 4*

1 tablespoon extra-virgin olive oil

3 fennel bulbs, trimmed of feathery stalks and quartered

1¼ cups reduced-sodium vegetable broth

Juice of 1 medium orange

¼ cup pitted oil-cured black olives

¼ teaspoon kosher salt

¼ teaspoon freshly ground black pepper

1 tablespoon unsalted butter

Heat the olive oil in a large sauté pan or skillet over high heat. Add the fennel, cut-sides down. Cook, undisturbed, until the fennel browns, 2 to 3 minutes. Add the broth, orange juice, olives, salt, and pepper. Cover with a lid and reduce the heat to medium-low so the liquid is still heartily simmering. Cook until the fennel is tender, 20 to 25 minutes. Transfer the fennel to a plate, then increase the heat to high. Let the liquid boil until it reduces significantly, about 2 minutes. Remove from the heat, add the butter, stir to melt, and pour over the fennel.

DO THE DASH   For a mere 27 calories for a 1-cup serving, fennel is a good source of fiber, potassium, and vitamin C. Plus, research suggests consuming stronger-flavored items like fennel, radishes, and arugula can leave you feeling satisfied with less overall calorie intake.

SHOPPING TIP   Don't compost the green stalks from your fennel. They can make a nutritious addition to stir-fries, soups, and homemade veggie stock.

NUTRITION   Per Serving: 135 calories; 2 grams protein; 16 grams carbohydrate; 6 grams fiber; 8 grams fat (2 grams saturated); 353 mg sodium

Cilantro Brown Rice

Brown rice is very healthy, but often makes for a pretty boring side dish on its lonesome. Here, brown rice is given a huge boost of flavor from cilantro, scallions, lime, and avocado. Even better, enhancing the flavor is hardly any work at all. *SERVES 4*

1 cup brown rice	Juice of 1 lime
1 bunch cilantro leaves, washed	1 clove garlic, crushed
1 avocado, chopped (see page 137)	½ teaspoon kosher salt
2 scallions, coarsely chopped	1 tablespoon extra-virgin olive oil

In a medium pot, cook the brown rice according to the package instructions. When the rice is almost done, puree the cilantro, avocado, scallions, lime juice, garlic, and salt in a food processor. Pour the olive oil through the feed tube and puree until smooth, 1 to 2 minutes. When the rice is tender, drain, and return to the pot. Add the cilantro seasoning to the rice, and stir to combine.

DO THE DASH Studies have shown that brown rice generates a lower glycemic response in the body than white rice does, meaning that it causes less of a spike in blood sugar. This trait may be beneficial in the dietary management of chronic diseases such as diabetes and heart disease.

SHOPPING TIP Scooping up your brown rice from bulk bins can often save you money versus buying it already packaged.

NUTRITION Per Serving: 288 calories; 5 grams protein; 42 grams carbohydrate; 5 grams fiber; 12 grams fat (2 grams saturated); 300 mg sodium

PASTA

Who doesn't enjoy sitting down to a plateful of pasta? It's versatile and affordable, and feels like a complete meal in one dish. Pick a pasta shape, a protein, and a vegetable and meld the components into a meal. Pasta has become a global food, so you can pull flavors from any continent into a pasta dish. Tomatoes combine with chickpeas and spices for an Indian flair; soy sauce, snow peas, and sesame oil mix together in an Asian homage to pasta salad. And whether you make a baked pasta dish that slowly melds the flavors together or a quickly cooked one that picks up the bright flavors around it, pasta is all about tying together an array of savors. The DASH Diet strongly recommends swapping out refined grains for more nutrient-dense whole ones, so try to select whole grain pastas for these recipes when possible. While I believe the pasta selected in each recipe works well with recommended sauces and other ingredients, feel free to make substitutions. If you're not a fan of capellini but love fettuccine, follow your heart—that's what cooking is about.

Fettucine with Lemon Shrimp

Shrimp doesn't need a lot of assistance. This simple dish of pasta, shrimp, lemon, and cheese has a somewhat indulgent simplicity.   *SERVES 6*

1 pound whole grain fettuccine

3½ tablespoons extra-virgin olive oil, plus more as needed

Grated zest and juice of 2 lemons

½ cup grated Parmigiano-Reggiano cheese

1 (16-ounce) bag frozen uncooked shrimp, thawed

¼ teaspoon kosher salt

¼ teaspoon freshly ground black pepper

2 cloves garlic, minced

Cook the pasta in large pot of boiling salted water until tender but still firm to the bite, stirring occasionally. Meanwhile, make the lemon sauce: In a medium bowl, combine 3 tablespoons of the olive oil, lemon zest, lemon juice, and cheese. Set aside. Drain the pasta in a colander, reserving ¼ cup pasta water, return the pasta to the pot, toss with a drizzle of olive oil, and keep hot.

Season the shrimp with salt and pepper. Heat the remaining ½ tablespoon olive oil in a large sauté pan or skillet over medium-high heat. Add the shrimp and garlic and sauté until the shrimp is pink, 2 to 3 minutes. Remove from the heat. Add the reserved pasta and pasta water to the pan with the shrimp along with the lemon sauce, stirring to mix. Taste, and adjust the seasonings as needed.

DO THE DASH   Shrimp are one of the few foods that contain a decent amount of vitamin D. On top of its bone-building efficiency, vitamin D has been shown to reduce the risk of several diseases like certain cancers and heart disease.

SHOPPING TIP   When possible, select farmed or wild-caught shrimp from North America which is a more sustainable choice than the imported shrimp which currently dominates the market.

NUTRITION   Per Serving: 450 calories; 29 grams protein; 52 grams carbohydrate; 2 grams fiber; 13 grams fat (3 grams saturated); 341 mg sodium

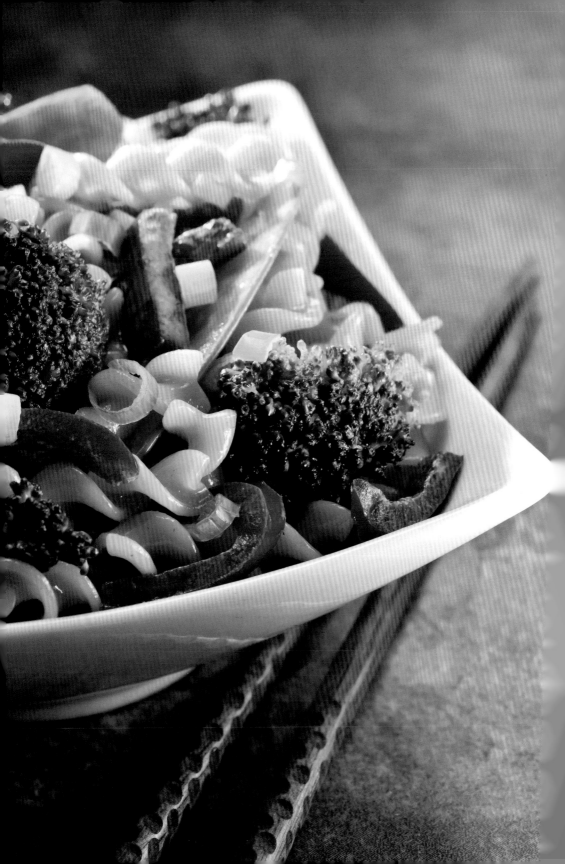

Asian-Style Pasta Salad

This pasta salad is a big hit every time I make it. It's great as an appetizer or as lunch, but can also be a light warm-weather entrée. *SERVES 6*

1 pound whole-wheat fusilli or other shaped pasta

3 tablespoons sesame oil

2 tablespoons honey

2 tablespoons reduced-sodium soy sauce

2 tablespoons balsamic vinegar

½ cup low-fat mayonnaise

¼ teaspoon kosher salt

¼ teaspoon freshly ground black pepper

1 teaspoon canola oil

2 red bell peppers, chopped

1½ cup broccoli florets

2 cups snow peas

3 scallions, thinly sliced

1 tablespoon sesame seeds

Cook the pasta in large pot of boiling salted water until tender but still firm to the bite, stirring occasionally. Drain very well. Transfer to large bowl. In a small bowl, whisk the sesame oil, honey, soy sauce, vinegar, mayonnaise, salt, and pepper until blended. Mix half of the dressing into the pasta. Heat the canola oil in a heavy large sauté pan or skillet over medium-high heat. Add the bell peppers and broccoli, cooking until just wilted, about 5 minutes. Add the snow peas and toss with the vegetables. Sauté until the snow peas are tender, just 1 minute. Add the vegetable mixture to the pasta. Add the remaining dressing, stirring to combine. Garnish with the scallions and sesame seeds, and serve at room temperature.

DO THE DASH   Studies show that if you beef up dishes such as this one with plenty of bulky vegetables like broccoli, you'll be satisfied with less calorie intake, which could help with weight loss and, subsequently, blood pressure reduction. So this dish should easily provide 6 servings.

SHOPPING TIP   When shopping for dry pastas, make sure the first ingredient is a whole grain such as whole wheat, spelt, or kamut.

NUTRITION   Per Serving: 472 calories; 14 grams protein; 72 grams carbohydrate; 3 grams fiber; 17 grams fat (2 grams saturated); 425 mg sodium

Spaghetti and Meatballs

Turkey and extra-lean beef are combined in a compromise that delivers a less fatty meatball full of rich, meaty flavor. *SERVES 4*

1 pound whole wheat spaghetti
½ pound ground turkey breast
½ pound extra-lean ground beef
½ teaspoon kosher salt
¼ teaspoon freshly ground pepper
2 teaspoons Worcestershire sauce

1 large egg
¼ cup panko bread crumbs
1 tablespoon dried parsley flakes
1 (25-ounce) jar marinara sauce
1 tablespoon unsalted butter

Cook the pasta in large pot of boiling salted water until tender but still firm to the bite, stirring occasionally. Drain in a colander, reserving ¼ cup pasta water, toss with a drizzle of olive oil, and reserve.

Make the meatballs: Preheat the oven to 425°F. Line a rimmed baking sheet with foil, and spray the foil with cooking spray. In a large bowl, combine the turkey, beef, salt, pepper, Worcestershire sauce, egg, bread crumbs, and parsley. Using a spoon or your hands, mix until combined. Form each meatball by rolling about 1 tablespoon of the mixture into a ball and placing on the prepared baking sheet. You should have about 30 meatballs. Bake until cooked through, about 15 minutes.

Meanwhile, heat the marinara sauce and butter in a large pot over medium-high heat. Let simmer so the flavors mingle, about 10 minutes. When the meatballs are ready, add to the sauce, and let cook 5 minutes longer. Add the reserved pasta. Thin the sauce with the reserved pasta water if needed. Simmer until the pasta is hot, and serve.

DO THE DASH Cooked tomato products like marinara sauce are a fantastic source of the heart-healthy antioxidant lycopene. Just make sure you compare the sodium levels in several brands before purchasing one.

SHOPPING TIP Coarsely ground Japanese-style panko bread crumbs are crispier and crunchier than their Western counterparts, making them a worthwhile upgrade.

NUTRITION Per Serving: 502 calories; 37 grams protein; 59 grams carbohydrate; 10 grams fiber; 13 grams fat (5 grams saturated); 506 mg sodium

Zucchini Pesto with Capellini

Pesto doesn't need to be made with basil—zucchini does double-duty in this recipe: Grated, sautéed zucchini is featured, and raw zucchini is used for the pesto. Light and fresh, this pasta feels like summer any time of year. *SERVES 4*

1 pound whole-grain capellini, or other thin pasta

⅓ cup plus 2 teaspoons extra-virgin olive oil

4 medium to large zucchini, divided

2 medium cloves garlic, smashed

½ cup unsalted walnuts

½ cup grated Parmigiano-Reggiano cheese

¼ teaspoon kosher salt

¼ teaspoon freshly ground pepper

Cook the pasta in a large pot of boiling salted water until tender but still firm to the bite, stirring occasionally. Drain in a colander, reserving ¼ cup pasta water, toss with a little olive oil, and reserve.

Meanwhile, make the pesto: Coarsely chop 1½ of the zucchini and put in a food processor. Add the garlic, walnuts, cheese, salt, and pepper and puree. Pour ⅓ cup of the olive oil through the feed tube, and puree until the mixture is emulsified. Add more oil if necessary.

Position a box grater in a large bowl, and grate the remaining 2½ zucchini. Heat the remaining 2 teaspoons olive oil in a large sauté pan or skillet over medium-high heat. Add the grated zucchini and season with salt and pepper. Sauté the zucchini until tender, 3 to 5 minutes. Reduce the heat to low and add the reserved pasta, pasta water, and pesto, stirring to combine. Simmer until the pasta is hot. Taste, adjust the seasonings as needed, and serve.

DO THE DASH   Among nuts, walnuts contain the most omega-3 fatty acids, making them a champion for heart health. Add them to salads and oatmeal or use in lieu of more expensive pine nuts when making pesto.

SHOPPING TIP   For the best flavor (and value!), buy a chunk of Parmigiano-Reggiano cheese and grate as needed.

NUTRITION   Per Serving: 427 calories; 15 grams protein; 39 grams carbohydrate; 8 grams fiber; 26 grams fat (5 grams saturated); 360 mg sodium

Spinach-Stuffed Shells

Tofu is oh-so-subtly added to these shells to give your diet an added protein boost without all the fat of excess cheese. *SERVES 6*

¾ (12-ounce) box jumbo pasta shells, preferably whole grain

2 teaspoons extra-virgin olive oil

14 ounces soft tofu, chopped

1 large egg

12 ounces fresh mozzarella, shredded, divided

½ teaspoon kosher salt

½ teaspoon freshly ground black pepper

1 teaspoon garlic powder

1 tablespoon dried parsley flakes

1 (25-ounce) jar marinara sauce, preferably low sodium, divided

½ (16-ounce) package frozen chopped spinach, thawed

Cook the pasta in a large pot of boiling salted water until tender but still firm to the bite, stirring occasionally. Drain in a colander, drizzle with the olive oil, and reserve. Make the spinach stuffing: In a large bowl, combine the tofu, egg, half of the mozzarella, salt, pepper, garlic powder, parsley flakes, and ¾ cup of the marinara sauce. Squeeze the excess liquid from the spinach, add to the bowl, and mix.

Preheat the oven to 350°F. Place the reserved pasta shells in a 9 x 13-inch baking dish. Using a spoon, fill each shell with spinach stuffing. When finished, sprinkle the remaining cheese on the shells, then pour the remaining marinara sauce on top. Bake until warmed through, about 30 minutes.

DO THE DASH Enjoy Meatless Mondays by embracing tofu. It's an excellent low-fat protein substitute to meat. In dishes such as this, it soaks up the surrounding flavors beautifully.

SHOPPING TIP When purchasing extra-virgin olive oils, make sure to choose only those packaged in dark bottles to help prevent any damage from the lighting in the store.

NUTRITION Per Serving: 547 calories; 30 grams protein; 65 grams carbohydrate; 5 grams fiber; 21 grams fat (9 grams saturated); 655 mg sodium

Linguine with Tomatoes and Eggplant

Use a nonstick pan for this recipe. Eggplants are like sponges, they'll just keep soaking up all the olive oil that you use, so it's healthier and easier to use a nonstick pan. *SERVES 4*

1½ teaspoons olive oil

2 medium eggplants, peeled and chopped into small pieces

1 (25-ounce) jar marinara sauce, preferably low sodium

¼ teaspoon kosher salt

¼ teaspoon freshly ground black pepper

1 pound whole wheat linguine

Grated Parmigiano-Reggiano cheese (optional)

Make the sauce: Heat the olive oil in a large nonstick sauté pan or skillet over medium-high heat. Add the eggplant, and cook, stirring occasionally, until slightly soft, 10 to 12 minutes. Add the marinara sauce and stir to combine with the eggplant. Reduce the heat to low, cover the pan, and let simmer until the eggplant pieces are soft, 30 to 35 minutes. Season with the salt and pepper.

Meanwhile, cook the pasta in a large pot of boiling salted water until tender but still firm to the bite, stirring occasionally. Drain in a colander. Add the pasta to the sauce, and heat until the pasta is hot. Top with cheese, if using, or pass at the table.

DO THE DASH   The DASH diet recommends 6 to 8 servings of grains a day and at least half of these should be more nutrient-packed whole grains such as the linguine used in this recipe.

SHOPPING TIP   You can now find various kinds of whole-grain linguine and other pastas, such as spelt or kamut, that offer different flavors and nutritional perks. As they say, "Variety is the spice of life."

NUTRITION   Per Serving: 372 calories; 12 grams protein; 70 grams carbohydrate; 19 grams fiber; 8 grams fat (2 grams saturated); 207 mg sodium

11/27/2016

Turkey Lasagne

Garfield isn't the only one who loves lasagne. This turkey-based version of the popular Italian staple is great for a big crowd or to give yourself a couple days of leftovers. SERVES 8

2 teaspoons canola oil

1 pound extra-lean ground turkey breast

½ teaspoon kosher salt

¼ teaspoon freshly ground black pepper

1 (25-ounce) jar tomato sauce

1 (15-ounce) container low-fat ricotta cheese

1 large egg

½ cup shredded zucchini

½ cup shredded carrot

1 (16-ounce) box no-boil whole wheat lasagna noodles (12 noodles will be needed)

1 (12-ounce) package part-skim shredded mozzarella cheese

Preheat the oven to 375°F. Heat the canola oil in a medium saucepan over medium-high heat. Add the ground turkey, salt, and pepper and sauté, stirring occasionally, until the turkey is fully cooked, about 8 minutes. Remove from the heat and stir in three-fourths of the pasta sauce. In a medium bowl, combine the ricotta, egg, zucchini, carrot, and remaining pasta sauce.

Add 1 to 2 tablespoons ricotta sauce to a 9 x 13-inch glass baking dish. Top with 4 noodles and all but 1 cup of the turkey sauce. Sprinkle 1 cup mozzarella cheese on top of the sauce. Layer with 4 more noodles. Add all but 1 cup of the ricotta sauce and top with 4 noodles. Combine the remaining ricotta sauce and turkey sauce and spread over the noodles. Sprinkle the remaining mozzarella on top. Cover the dish with foil and bake until the noodles are easily pierced with a knife, about 45 minutes. Remove the foil and cook for 15 minutes longer, until the cheese is golden. Cut the lasagne into serving pieces.

DO THE DASH   When making pasta based dishes such as lasagne, make sure to sneak in as many vegetables as possible such as the carrots and zucchini in this recipe. In a recent Pennsylvania State University study, adults who consumed meals that incorporated additional vegetables took in up to 357 fewer calories a day and almost doubled their intake of veggies.

Yum! Next time, we'll make it w/o the turkey and w/more veggies! —An

VERY GOOD.
DOESN'T NEED MEAT.
~JS

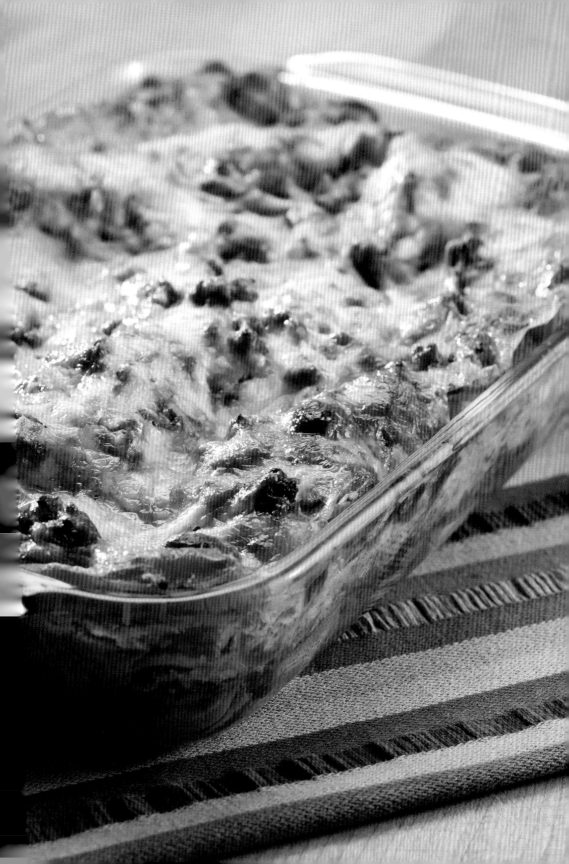

SHOPPING TIP Lasagne can be anything but low in calories, so you'll want to make sure to shop for lower-fat versions of items such as ground meat, ricotta cheese, and mozzarella cheese.

NUTRITION Per Serving: 518 calories; 41 grams protein; 56 grams carbohydrate; 10 grams fiber; 17 grams fat (8 grams saturated); 539 mg sodium

Spaghetti with Eggs and Ramps

Ramps are an early spring vegetable, beloved along the East Coast. This dish highlights their exciting flavor, but if you're really in the mood and it's not ramp season, any equal amount of scallions or a dozen garlic scapes are a good substitute. *SERVES 4*

1 pound whole wheat linguine

3½ tablespoons extra-virgin olive oil, divided

25 to 30 ramps, greens and whites separated

4 large eggs

⅓ cup grated Parmigiano-Reggiano cheese

Cook the pasta in a large pot of boiling salted water until tender but still firm to the bite, stirring occasionally. Drain in a colander, reserving ½ cup pasta water, toss with 1 tablespoon olive oil, and reserve.

In a large nonstick sauté pan or skillet, heat 2½ tablespoons of the olive oil. Add the ramp whites. Cook, stirring occasionally, until fragrant, 1 to 2 minutes. Add the eggs and fry until the whites are set (without flipping). Remove from the heat. Add the ramp greens, reserved pasta water, and pasta. Stir until the pasta is hot and well-coated with egg yolk. Garnish with cheese.

DO THE DASH When possible, seek out fruits and vegetables such as ramps that are in season locally since they will be at their flavor and nutrient peak.

SHOPPING TIP An excellent place to find a wide assortment of in-season produce at reasonable prices is at your local farmers' market. Find one near you at www.localharvest.org.

NUTRITION Per Serving: 380 calories; 17 grams protein; 37 grams carbohydrate; 7 grams fiber; 20 grams fat (5 grams saturated); 215 mg sodium

Angel Hair with Tomatoes and Chickpeas

With cumin, coriander, and cardamom, this pasta dish delivers an Indian spin on an Italian tomato sauce. If you want to rely entirely on pantry staples, you can substitute 1 tablespoon of dried basil for the fresh variety and make this dish without another trip to the store.   *SERVES 6*

2 tablespoons extra-virgin olive oil

2 cloves garlic, minced

1 tablespoon ground cumin

1 tablespoon ground coriander

½ teaspoon ground cardamom *(nutmeg/ cinnamon)*

¼ teaspoon red pepper flakes

2 (15-ounce) cans chickpeas, rinsed and drained

1 (28-ounce) can peeled whole plum tomatoes, including juice

½ cup chopped fresh basil

¼ teaspoon kosher salt

¼ teaspoon freshly ground black pepper

1 pound capelli d'angelo (angel hair pasta)

Make the sauce: Heat the olive oil in a large sauté pan or skillet over medium heat. Add the garlic, cumin, coriander, cardamom, and pepper flakes, and stir constantly, until the oil is fragrant and somewhat darker, 1 to 2 minutes. Stir in the chickpeas. Add the tomatoes, breaking them up with a spoon. Simmer, stirring occasionally, until slightly thickened, about 20 minutes. Stir in the basil and season to taste with salt and pepper.

Meanwhile, cook the pasta in a large pot of boiling salted water until tender but still firm to the bite, stirring occasionally. Drain the pasta and serve with the sauce ladled over the top.

DO THE DASH   Chickpeas are a wonderful source of good stuff like fiber, blood pressure–lowering potassium, folate, and vitamin B6. If you want to further reduce your sodium intake, try soaking and boiling dried chickpeas instead of using canned.

SHOPPING TIP   Some brands like Eden Organic now offer "no salt added" canned beans.

NUTRITION   Per Serving: 444 calories; 17 grams protein; 79 grams carbohydrate; 10 grams fiber; 7 grams fat (1 gram saturated); 326 mg sodium

Really like the flavor - need to thicken the sauce somehow. -ch

GOOD, BUT COULD USE SOME MORE FLAVOR.
- gs

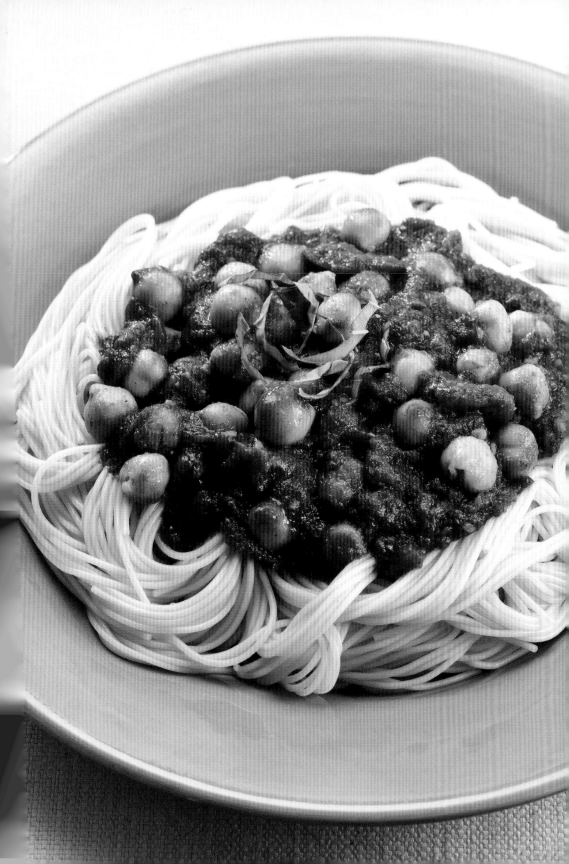

POULTRY

Poultry is a staple of the typical health-conscious carnivore's diet. A good source of protein and lower in fat than much of the beef and pork on the market, poultry is an easy choice. Purchasing organic, vegetarian-fed, antibiotic-free cuts of poultry means you can have your poultry and feel extra good about it. Of course, organic chicken costs a bit more, but there are still ways to save money.

First, buy dark meat instead of white, and enjoy the added benefit of extra flavor and moistness. Instead of purchasing pieces of chicken already butchered and trimmed of fat, buy a whole one, and ask your butcher to cut it into pieces for no extra cost. Also, read over grocery store flyers and their websites for sales, as they often have bargains on poultry. Or buy more than you need, and store it in the freezer for later use. Add the warmth of cinnamon and comfort of apples to the traditional roasted chicken, utilize the cheapness of turkey drumsticks for a homage-to-Thanksgiving meal, and let fruit salsa adorn and pep up the usual sautéed chicken breast.

Cinnamon-Scented Roasted Chicken with Apples

Cinnamon is known as a dessert ingredient but can also be a great addition to savory dishes. It adds warmth to this braised chicken. And here's a tip: Removing the backbone from the chicken shortens the cooking time. *Serves 4*

3 Red Delicious apples, sliced

2 tablespoons unsalted butter, at room temperature

2 teaspoons grated orange zest (about 1 orange)

1 teaspoon ground cinnamon

½ teaspoon kosher salt

¼ teaspoon freshly ground black pepper

1 (3¼ to 3½-pound) whole chicken

Preheat the oven to 425°F. Spread the apples in the baking dish. Combine the butter, orange zest, cinnamon, salt, and pepper in a small bowl. Rinse the chicken and blot dry. Using poultry shears or a knife, cut the backbone out. Place the chicken split-side down on top of the apples. Rub half of the butter mixture underneath the skin. Rub the remaining half on the skin. Roast the chicken until the thickest part of the thigh reaches 180°F or the juices run clear when pricked, about 40 minutes. Tent the chicken with aluminum foil to keep warm and let rest for about 5 minutes. Cut the chicken into pieces, and serve with the roasted apples and juices.

DO THE DASH Preparing a whole chicken is a great way to save money, but make sure to only enjoy a bite or two of the skin since this is where the majority of its saturated fat lies.

SHOPPING TIP The Environmental Working Group found that among fruits, apples can contain the most pesticide residues. So, when possible, splurge for organic.

NUTRITION Per Serving: 329 calories; 32 grams protein; 19 grams carbohydrate; 3 grams fiber; 14 grams fat (6 grams saturated); 387 mg sodium

Chicken with Jalapeño-Cilantro Sauce

Between the limey-cumin marinade that the chicken takes a soak in and the addition of a creamy Peruvian sauce spiked with jalapeño and cilantro, the chicken breasts are infused with plenty of flavor. SERVES 4

½ cup plus 1 teaspoon freshly squeezed lime juice

3½ tablespoons canola oil, divided

1½ teaspoons paprika

2 teaspoons ground cumin

4 skin-on, boneless chicken breasts (about 2½ pounds)

3 jalapeño chiles, seeded and coarsely chopped

1 cup loosely packed cilantro, coarsely chopped

1 clove garlic, crushed

⅓ cup low-fat mayonnaise

1 tablespoon water

¼ teaspoon kosher salt

¼ teaspoon freshly ground black pepper

Combine ½ cup of the lime juice, 2 tablespoons canola oil, paprika, and cumin in a small bowl. Put the chicken in a zippered bag, pour in the marinade, close securely, turn over and around to distribute the marinade, and put the bag in a bowl (in case of leakage). Refrigerate for 2 to 3 hours. Meanwhile, make the sauce: Combine the chiles, cilantro, garlic, mayonnaise, remaining lime juice, water, salt, and pepper to a food processor. Puree until smooth, 30 seconds to 1 minute. Taste and adjust the salt and lime juice as needed. Transfer to a container, and refrigerate until needed.

Preheat the oven to 400°F. Heat 1½ tablespoons canola oil in a large ovenproof sauté pan or skillet over high heat. Season the chicken with salt and pepper, and carefully add to the pan skin-side down. Cook the chicken until browned, about 8 minutes. Turn the chicken over, and cook another 2 minutes. Roast the chicken breasts in the oven to an internal temperature of 165°F, 15 to 20 minutes. Serve with the jalapeño-cilantro sauce.

DO THE DASH   Herbs such as cilantro are a great way to punch up the flavor of the dishes for very little caloric cost. Plus, most of them contain a range of beneficial antioxidants and nutrients like vitamin C, which has been shown to keep blood pressure numbers healthy. Remember: The chicken skin adds flavor during the cooking process, but is best to remove before eating to save on calories.

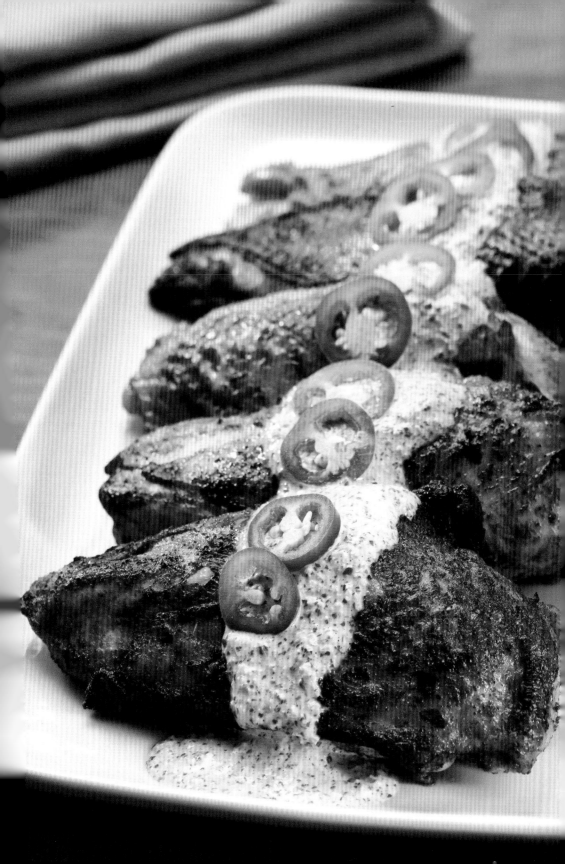

SHOPPING TIP The best flavor comes from squeezing fresh limes or lemons for their juice as opposed to buying pre-made bottled juice.

NUTRITION Per Serving: 324 calories; 28 grams protein; 5 grams carbohydrate; 1 gram fiber; 21 grams fat (2 grams saturated); 376 mg sodium

Braised Chipotle Turkey Drumsticks with Sweet Potatoes

Pound per pound, turkey drumsticks are a lot cheaper than chicken. Like most cheaper meats, they do require a longer cooking time, but it's all unattended. Pair this with the couscous and dried cranberries on page 49 as an ode to the Thanksgiving meal. *Serves 4*

1 tablespoon canola oil

3 (1-pound) turkey drumsticks

¼ teaspoon kosher salt

1 medium yellow onion, chopped

4 cloves garlic, smashed

2 cups reduced-sodium chicken broth

1 canned chipotle chile plus 2 teaspoons adobo sauce

¼ teaspoon freshly ground black pepper

3 medium sweet potatoes

1 tablespoon flour

1 tablespoon unsalted butter, at room temperature

Heat the canola oil in a large Dutch oven over medium-high heat. Season the drumsticks with the salt. Brown for 3 to 4 minutes on each side. Transfer the drumsticks to a platter. Add the onion to the pot and cook, stirring occasionally, until slightly softened, 2 to 3 minutes. Add the garlic and cook 1 minute, then add the chicken broth, chipotle chile, adobo sauce, and pepper. Bring to a boil, then return the turkey to the pot. Cover with a lid, reduce the heat to low, and simmer for 1 hour. Meanwhile, peel the sweet potatoes, and chop into 1-inch cubes. In a small bowl, combine the flour and the butter, and place in the freezer.

Turn the drumsticks over. Continue cooking, and after 40 minutes longer, add the sweet potatoes. Cook until the turkey and the sweet potatoes are very tender, about 20 minutes longer. Transfer the turkey and the sweet potatoes to a platter, and tent with foil to keep warm. Carefully remove the chile and all but 1½ cups of the broth from the pot. Turn the heat to high, whisk in the reserved butter and flour mixture, and boil until the sauce is as thick as you desire, a few minutes. While the sauce is reducing, carve the turkey. When the sauce is ready, pour over the turkey and sweet potatoes, and serve.

DO THE DASH Turkey meat is a good source of selenium, a mineral which is incorporated into proteins to make selenoproteins that are important antioxidant enzymes in the body.

SHOPPING TIP   You can find chipotle chiles in adobo sauce in the Latin section of most grocery stores. It adds a wonderful smoky heat to dishes.

NUTRITION   Per Serving: 303 calories; 24 grams protein; 27 grams carbohydrate; 4 grams fiber; 11 grams fat (4 grams saturated); 560 mg sodium

Chicken and Rice with Ginger Sauce

It sounds simple, but there's something intricately delicious about chicken and rice. Add a gingery sauce to pour over the chicken and stir into the rice, and magic happens. Note: The knobbiness of the ginger makes it hard to use a peeler to remove the brown peel. An easier way is to use a spoon to scrape the peel away. *SERVES 4*

⅓ cup canola oil plus 2 teaspoons, divided

1½ pounds boneless, skinless chicken thighs

½ teaspoon kosher salt, divided

3 cups water plus 3 tablespoons, divided

1½ cups uncooked brown basmati rice

½ pound fresh ginger, peeled and cut into pieces

Heat 2 teaspoons of the canola oil in a large heavy pot over high heat. Season the chicken thighs with ¼ teaspoon of the salt and sauté just 2 to 3 minutes on each side, in batches if needed (browning isn't necessary). Transfer the chicken to a plate. Add 3 cups of the water, stirring to incorporate any bits on the bottom of the pot. Add the rice and bring to a boil. Return the chicken to the pot, and cover with a lid. Reduce the heat to low, and simmer until the rice is tender, about 20 minutes. Remove from the heat and let sit 10 minutes.

Meanwhile, make the ginger sauce: In a food processor, puree the ginger, remaining 3 tablespoons water, and remaining ¼ teaspoon salt while pouring the remaining ⅓ cup canola oil down the feed tube. Puree until emulsified. Taste the sauce, and adjust the seasoning if needed. Serve the chicken and rice with generous portions of ginger sauce.

DO THE DASH Findings, recently published in the American Journal of Clinical Nutrition, determined that people who regularly eat whole grains such as brown rice rather than refined grains like white rice pack on less visceral adipose tissue—the fat that surrounds the intra-abdominal organs that has been linked to a higher risk for heart disease and type 2 diabetes.

SHOPPING TIP Bulk bins at supermarkets are a great place to find whole grains like brown rice in quantities that you can control.

NUTRITION Per Serving: 675 calories; 40 grams protein; 64 grams carbohydrate; 4 grams fiber; 29 grams fat (4 grams saturated); 447 mg sodium

Orange-Glazed Chicken over Spinach

Orange marmalade does all the work for you, creating the sauce for this glazed chicken. Add a little spinach for a quick and healthy meal. *SERVES 4*

1 tablespoon canola oil, divided

1 (9-ounce) bag spinach

½ teaspoon kosher salt, divided

½ teaspoon freshly ground black pepper, divided

1½ pounds chicken cutlets

½ cup orange marmalade

2 tablespoons pure maple syrup

Juice of 1 lemon

1 tablespoon sodium reduced soy sauce

1 teaspoon poppy seeds

1 tablespoon almond slivers, for garnish

Heat 1½ teaspoons of the canola oil in a large sauté pan or skillet over medium high heat. Add half the spinach, and season with ¼ teaspoon of the salt and ¼ teaspoon of the pepper. Cook the spinach, stirring, until almost wilted, 2 to 3 minutes. Add the remaining spinach, and continue to cook, stirring again, until all the spinach is wilted, about 3 more minutes. Cover with a lid to keep warm, remove from the heat, and set aside.

Wipe the pan clean and heat the remaining 1½ teaspoons canola oil over high heat. Season the chicken cutlets with the remaining ¼ teaspoon each salt and pepper, and add to the pan. Sauté until the chicken is golden, 2 to 3 minutes. Flip the chicken over and cook on the second side until golden, 2 to 3 minutes longer. Meanwhile, make the orange sauce: In a small bowl, whisk the orange marmalade, maple syrup, lemon juice, soy sauce, and poppy seeds until combined. When the chicken is golden, add the orange sauce to the pan. Using tongs, coat the chicken with the sauce, letting the sauce reduce, until the chicken is well glazed, 2 to 3 minutes. Remove from the heat. Use a paper towel to blot any excess liquid from the spinach. Divide the spinach among serving plates and top with the chicken. Pour the sauce over the chicken and serve garnished with almond slivers.

DO THE DASH Naturally occurring nitrates in leafy greens like spinach have been shown to help reduce blood pressure numbers by improving artery dilation.

SHOPPING TIP Chicken cutlets are boneless chicken breasts that have been pounded very thin. They cook very quickly, making them a great choice for a speedy weeknight dinner.

NUTRITION Per Serving: 375 calories; 42 grams protein; 38 grams carbohydrate; 2 grams fiber; 7 grams fat (1 gram saturated); 612 mg sodium

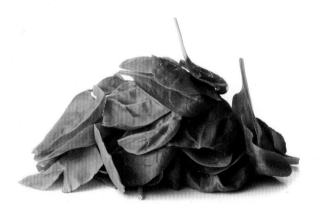

VERY GOOD STUFF, ESPECIALLY THE GLAZE. SERVE OVER RICE, COULD ADD MUSHROOMS/ONIONS.

-SS

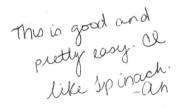

This is good and pretty easy. I like spinach. -an

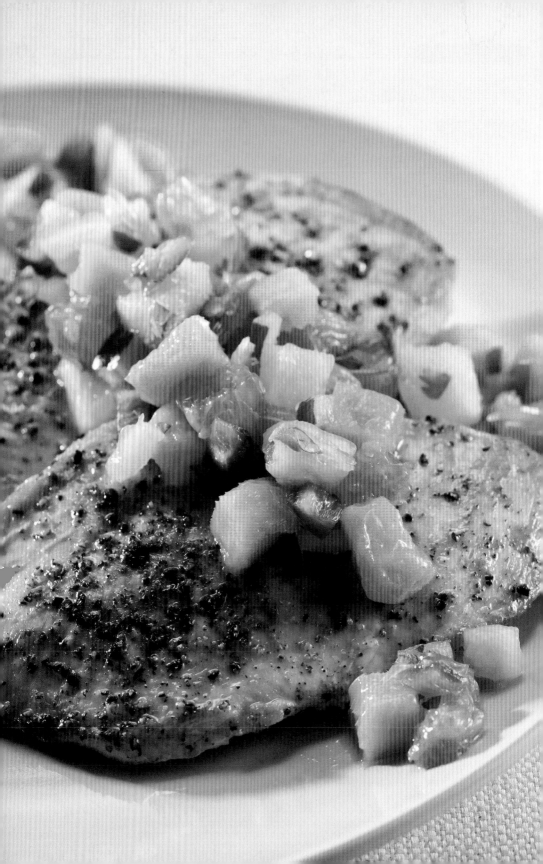

Chicken Cutlets with Fruit Salsa

Chicken tenders get a flavorful makeover from a tangy fruit salsa. *SERVES 6*

2 Ruby Red grapefruits

1 cup chopped pineapple

1 mango, chopped (see page 137)

¼ cup sliced red onion

1 to 3 jalapeño chiles, seeded and chopped

¼ cup chopped cilantro

½ teaspoon kosher salt, divided

¼ teaspoon freshly ground black pepper

1½ pounds chicken breast tenders

2 teaspoons canola oil

Make the salsa: Supreme the grapefruits into a large bowl (see page 138) and cut into bite-size pieces. Add the pineapple, mango, onion, jalapeño, cilantro, and ¼ teaspoon of the salt, and stir to combine. Set aside. Season the chicken tenders with remaining ¼ teaspoon salt and the pepper. Heat the canola oil in a medium sauté pan or skillet over medium-high heat. Working in batches if necessary, add the chicken and sauté until golden on one side, 2 to 3 minutes. Flip the chicken over and cook on the second side until golden, 2 to 3 minutes longer. Cut into the thickest piece to determine that it's no longer pink. Serve the chicken tenders with fruit salsa spooned over.

DO THE DASH   Homemade salsas are a great way to sneak more fruits and vegetables into mealtime. A great place to start is with grapefruit, which harbors blood pressure–lowering potassium.

SHOPPING TIP   Look for bags of cubed frozen mango in the freezer section of grocery stores, a convenient choice when fresh is not available.

NUTRITION   Per Serving: 389 calories; 18 grams protein; 37 grams carbohydrate; 4 grams fiber; 19 grams fat (4 grams saturated); 502 mg sodium

Scallion-Marinated Chicken

This scallion-heavy marinade pays homage to jerk flavors with a touch of allspice and thyme plus the heat of jalapeño. *SERVES 4*

2 bunches scallions, trimmed and coarsely chopped

2 jalapeño chiles, seeded and coarsely chopped

1½ tablespoons ground allspice

2 teaspoons dried thyme

4 cloves garlic

Juice of 1 lime

1 tablespoon reduced-sodium soy sauce

¼ cup plus 1 tablespoon canola oil, divided

1½ pounds boneless, skinless chicken thighs

¼ teaspoon kosher salt

¼ teaspoon freshly ground black pepper

In a food processor, add the scallions, jalapeños, allspice, thyme, garlic, lime juice, soy sauce, and ¼ cup of the canola oil. Puree until smooth, about 1 minute. Reserve ¼ cup of the marinade for basting. Pour the remaining marinade into a shallow dish and add the chicken thighs. Cover and refrigerate for 3 to 4 hours.

Preheat the oven to 400°F. Heat the remaining 1 tablespoon canola oil in a medium ovenproof sauté pan or skillet over medium-high heat. Season the chicken thighs with the salt and pepper, and sauté until brown, about 5 minutes. Using tongs, flip the chicken thighs over and cook until brown, 4 to 5 minutes longer. Roast the chicken, occasionally basting with the remaining marinade, until a meat thermometer registers 180°F, 10 to 15 minutes.

DO THE DASH When using scallions, make sure to include the green parts in recipes as they are a fantastic source of vitamin K, a necessary element for good bone health and proper blood clotting.

SHOPPING TIP For spices such as allspice that you may not use often, look in bulk bins. This way you can purchase smaller amounts and save money.

NUTRITION Per Serving: 226 calories; 34 grams protein; 6 grams carbohydrate; 2 grams fiber; 7 grams fat (2 grams saturated); 431 mg sodium

Chicken Marsala

Marsala is a sweet, inexpensive fortified wine that lends a ton of flavor to any fare, especially its namesake dish, where chicken and vegetables are simmered in a Marsala-heavy broth. Try serving alongside Polenta with Dried Mushrooms (page 39). Note: The combination of equal amounts of butter and flour is called *beurre manié,* French for "kneaded butter." It's used as a quick and easy way to thicken any sauce. *SERVES 4*

2 teaspoons canola oil

1 (10-ounce) container white mushrooms, halved

1 pint cherry tomatoes, halved

4 cloves garlic

1 cup reduced-sodium chicken broth

¾ cup Marsala

½ teaspoon kosher salt

¼ teaspoon freshly ground black pepper

1½ pounds chicken cutlets

1 tablespoon unsalted butter, at room temperature

1 tablespoon flour

Heat the canola oil in a large sauté pan or skillet over medium-high heat. Sauté the mushrooms and tomatoes, stirring occasionally, until the mushrooms are golden, 2 to 3 minutes. Add the garlic, and cook 1 minute. Add the chicken broth, Marsala, salt, and pepper, and use a spoon to scrape up any bits on the bottom. Bring the liquid to a boil. Nestle the chicken into the liquid, spooning the mushrooms and tomatoes on top of the chicken. Cover with a lid, and reduce the heat to low. Simmer the chicken until cooked through, 20 to 25 minutes. Cut into the thickest chicken piece to check for doneness.

Meanwhile, mix the butter and the flour in a small bowl. Put in the freezer to harden. Transfer the chicken from the pan into a serving dish. Bring the liquid to a boil over high heat. Add the butter and flour mixture, and whisk until the sauce thickens, 1 to 2 minutes, until it's as thick as you want. Taste and adjust the seasonings with salt and pepper as needed. Pour the sauce and vegetables over the chicken.

DO THE DASH Polysaccharide compounds in mushrooms are known for their immune-enhancing and anti-tumor properties.

SHOPPING TIP Chicken cutlets are thin pieces of chicken breast, which makes them very quick cooking. If you can't find them at your grocery store, simply pound chicken breasts with a kitchen mallet or heavy skillet between two pieces of plastic wrap to flatten.

NUTRITION   Per Serving: 310 calories; 43 grams protein; 8 grams carbohydrate; 1 grams fiber; 8 grams fat (3 grams saturated); 426 mg sodium

Asian-Style Chicken Thighs

Creating a spice blend like the Asian one in this recipe and then rubbing it underneath the skin of the chicken thighs before they're sautéed is a simple way to add tons of flavor to a chicken dish. *SERVES 4*

2 tablespoons grated fresh ginger

1 teaspoon ground cardamom

1 teaspoon ground cumin

Grated zest of 2 limes plus 1 teaspoon juice

½ teaspoon kosher salt

¼ teaspoon freshly ground black pepper

1½ tablespoons canola oil, divided

1½ pounds bone-in, skin-on chicken thighs

Preheat the oven to 400°F. Combine the ginger, cardamom, cumin, lime zest, lime juice, salt, pepper, and ½ tablespoon of the canola oil in a small bowl. Dividing the spice mixture evenly among the chicken pieces, use your fingers to lift the skin from the chicken and rub the spice underneath. Make sure to wipe off any spice mixture that isn't under the skin because it will burn. Season the outside of the chicken with salt and pepper. Heat the remaining 1 tablespoon canola oil in a medium nonstick ovenproof sauté pan or skillet over medium-high heat. Add the chicken thighs, skin-side down, and leave untouched to brown, 6 to 8 minutes. Using tongs, flip each chicken thigh over. Place skillet in the oven and roast until a meat thermometer registers 180°F, 10 to 15 minutes.

DO THE DASH   Preparing chicken meat with the skin and bone intact is a great way to lock in flavor. Just make sure to remove the skin before eating as it contains a high amount of saturated fat.

SHOPPING TIP   Many grocery stores offer discounts when buying cuts of chicken in bulk. So consider buying extra, and when you get home, divide the portions into zip-top bags for storage in the freezer.

NUTRITION   Per Serving (without skin): 399 calories; 44 grams protein; 0 grams carbohydrate; 0 grams fiber; 24 grams fat (5 grams saturated); 439 mg sodium

MEAT

Many health-conscious eaters avoid beef and pork, but in moderation, all foods can be part of a healthy DASH Diet. In fact, Australian researchers found that people following a low-sodium diet that also included lean red meat experienced drops in blood pressure. The USDA defines a lean cut of beef as a 3.5-ounce serving that contains less than 10 grams total fat, 4.5 grams saturated fat, and 95 milligrams cholesterol. Cuts of beef that meet these guidelines include: round cuts such as eye of round, top round, or bottom round; top sirloin and other loin cuts; flank steak; and extra-lean ground beef. But beware of the pitfalls when buying.

Meat that has already been marinated or assembled (like kebabs or stuffed chops) comes at a much higher price tag and can be pumped full of salt. Buy plain meat, and prepare it yourself. Also, rely on cheaper cuts of meat, like chuck roast and veal shoulder. If you splurge on the more expensive cuts, incorporate the meat into a dish with many other ingredients, like fajitas, to stretch the meat for more servings. And supplement meat-based dishes with plenty of extra vegetables. The DASH Diet recommends limiting your daily intake of meat to about 6 ounces, which leaves you caloric room for whole grains, healthy fats, and low-fat dairy products.

Meatloaf

This meatloaf is still comfort-worthy even with a healthier spin using lean ground beef and an abundance of grated veggies. This is just begging to be served with Buttermilk Mashed Potatoes (page 46). *SERVES 4*

2 small rolls (like brioche), torn into small pieces

¼ cup skim milk

2 tablespoons ketchup

2 teaspoons Worcestershire sauce

1 large zucchini, shredded

1 large carrot, shredded

1 large yellow squash, shredded

1 clove garlic, minced

1 pound lean ground sirloin

1 large egg

½ teaspoon kosher salt

½ teaspoon freshly ground black pepper

Preheat the oven to 350°F. Coat an 8 x 4-inch loaf pan with cooking spray. In a large bowl, combine the bread and the milk, and let sit for 5 minutes. Squeeze the milk from the bread, discarding the milk. Return the bread to the bowl, and add the ketchup, Worcestershire sauce, zucchini, carrot, squash, garlic, beef, egg, salt, and pepper. Using a spoon or your hands, combine the meat mixture well, but do not overmix. Transfer to the prepared pan. Bake until meatloaf is cooked through, 50 minutes to 1 hour.

DO THE DASH Dishes such as meatloaf are an opportunity to fortify them with an abundance of offerings from the produce aisle. This makes it easier to reach your daily vegetable quota.

SHOPPING TIP If you want the best flavor and freshest product, ask your butcher if they can grind up a sirloin steak on the spot with the excess fat trimmed off. Like other loin cuts, sirloin is considered a lean cut of beef.

NUTRITION Per Serving: 239 calories; 29 grams protein; 15 grams carbohydrate; 2 grams fiber; 7 grams fat (2 grams saturated); 474 mg sodium

Beef Fajitas with Red Peppers and Onions

Sometimes we all get a hankering for steak. The best way to indulge in this craving without a lot of damage to the waistline or wallet is to incorporate steak in a recipe like fajitas, where it's bulked up with veggies. *SERVES 4*

Grated zest and juice of 2 limes

2 tablespoons olive oil

3 cloves garlic, smashed

1¼ teaspoons ground cumin, divided

1 pound skirt steak

1 tablespoon canola oil

3 medium yellow onions, sliced

3 red bell peppers, sliced

¼ teaspoon kosher salt

¼ teaspoon freshly ground black pepper

¼ teaspoon cayenne pepper (optional)

8 (8-inch) whole wheat tortillas

1 avocado, sliced

Combine the lime zest and juice, olive oil, garlic, and 1 teaspoon of the cumin in a shallow dish. Add the steak and turn over in the marinade to cover. Cover and refrigerate for 1 to 2 hours, no more (the acid in the lime juice will make the meat mushy).

Heat the canola oil in a large sauté pan or skillet over medium-high heat. Add the onion, and cook, stirring occasionally, just until translucent, about 5 minutes. Add the bell pepper, salt, black pepper, cayenne pepper, and the remaining ¼ teaspoon cumin and stir to combine. Cook, stirring occasionally, until the onions are mostly caramelized and the bell peppers are cooked, about 10 minutes longer. Taste and adjust the seasonings as needed. Keep hot.

Preheat the broiler. Spread the tortillas on a rimmed baking sheet, and put in the oven to warm. Line a second rimmed baking sheet with foil. Remove the steak from the marinade and discard the marinade. Dab the steak with a paper towel to remove the excess marinade. Place on the prepared baking sheet and season with salt and pepper. Broil the steak about 4 minutes on each side, until it reaches medium-rare. Adjust the time for different thickness or doneness; if needed, make a cut into the center to determine doneness. Let the steak rest for 5 minutes, then cut across the grain into thin slices diagonally. Serve the steak and vegetables on the tortillas with avocado slices.

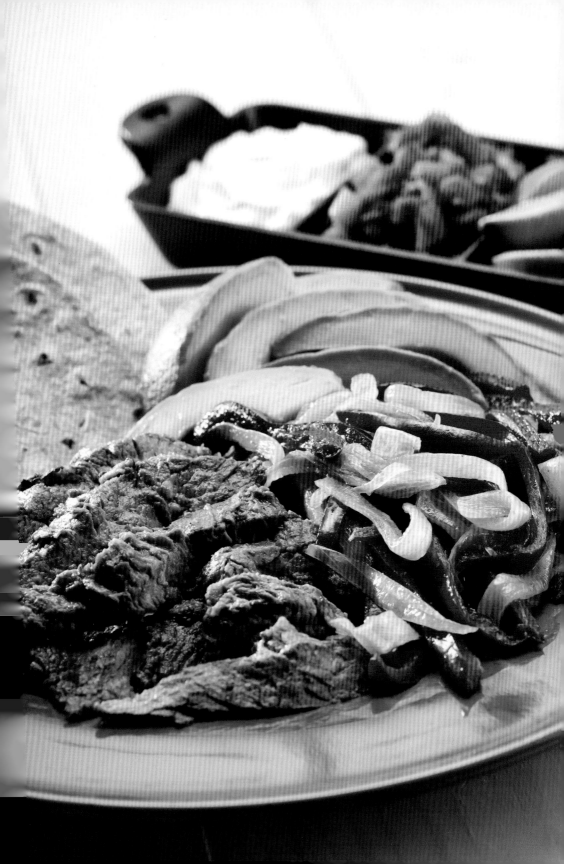

DO THE DASH   Compared to green bell peppers, the red variety contains nearly twice as much vitamin C and nine times more beta-carotene. In the body, beta-carotene is converted to vitamin A to help bolster bone, immune, and eye health.

SHOPPING TIP   When shopping for tortillas, make sure the first ingredient listed is a whole grain such as whole wheat flour as opposed to refined flour like white flour.

NUTRITION   Per Serving: 540 calories; 29 grams protein; 45 grams carbohydrate; 8 grams fiber; 28 grams fat (6 grams saturated); 374 mg sodium

Beef Tacos

I always seem to have a lingering jar of salsa in my fridge and a container of sour cream with just a dollop left in it. That's when it's taco time— pick up some taco shells and ground beef, and use up all those leftover condiments. Also, I tend to pile on grated carrots or any other produce I need to get rid of. *SERVES 4*

1 tablespoon flour
1 tablespoon chili powder
1 teaspoon ground turmeric
½ teaspoon ground cumin
2 teaspoons canola oil
1 pound extra-lean ground beef
¼ cup water

8 taco shells

Condiments:
6 to 8 radishes, chopped
2 tomatoes, chopped
1 cup shredded lettuce
Salsa, as needed

Combine the flour, chili powder, turmeric, and cumin in a small bowl. Heat the canola oil in a medium sauté pan or skillet over medium-high heat. Add the ground beef and sauté, stirring every couple of minutes to break up the meat, until the meat is browned and cooked, 6 to 7 minutes. Add the spice mixture and the water, and cook, stirring to coat the meat with the spices, until browned, 2 to 3 minutes. To serve, pile the meat into taco shells and let each guest add their own condiments.

DO THE DASH When buying an entire head of lettuce for a recipe like this that only calls for 1 cup of shredded lettuce, use the remaining lettuce for a side salad to get in extra veggies into your meal.

SHOPPING TIP If available in your supermarket, pick up a box of blue corn taco shells. Studies suggest that blue tinged corn has antioxidants similar to those found in blueberries and blackberries.

NUTRITION Per Serving: 329 calories; 28 grams protein; 24 grams carbohydrate; 3 grams fiber; 13 grams fat (4 grams saturated); 567 mg sodium

Skirt Steak in Lettuce Wraps with Pickled Vegetables

Lettuce serves as the wrap for broiled slices of skirt steak and quick-pickled veggies in this refreshing dish. *SERVES 4*

1 cup white vinegar
¼ cup sugar
1 bunch radishes, sliced
2 cucumbers, peeled and sliced
½ red onion, peeled and sliced

1 pound skirt steak
¼ teaspoon kosher salt
¼ teaspoon freshly ground black pepper
2 heads Boston lettuce, leaves separated

Make the pickled vegetables: Whisk the vinegar and the sugar in a small bowl until the sugar is mostly dissolved. Add the radishes, cucumbers, and onion, submerging in the vinegar, and let sit 15 to 20 minutes.

Preheat the broiler. Line a rimmed baking sheet with foil, and place the steak on the baking sheet. Season the steak with the salt and pepper. Broil to the desired doneness, about 3 minutes per side. Transfer to a work surface, and cover with a piece of foil. Let the steak rest for 5 minutes, then slice thinly across the grain, diagonally. To serve, place the pickled vegetables, lettuce leaves, and steak on a platter. Let everyone assemble their own wraps by filling lettuce cups with meat and vegetables.

DO THE DASH   Replacing wraps made with flour with those made with crisp lettuce leaves both trims calories and boosts your intake of vegetables.

SHOPPING TIP   There is an increasing trend among consumers to seek out "alternative" cuts of meat in the pursuit of slashing food bills. For example, skirt steak is a favorite choice for flavor, value, and versatility.

NUTRITION   Per Serving: 244 calories; 24 grams protein; 14 grams carbohydrate; 4 grams fiber; 9 grams fat (3 grams saturated); 223 mg sodium

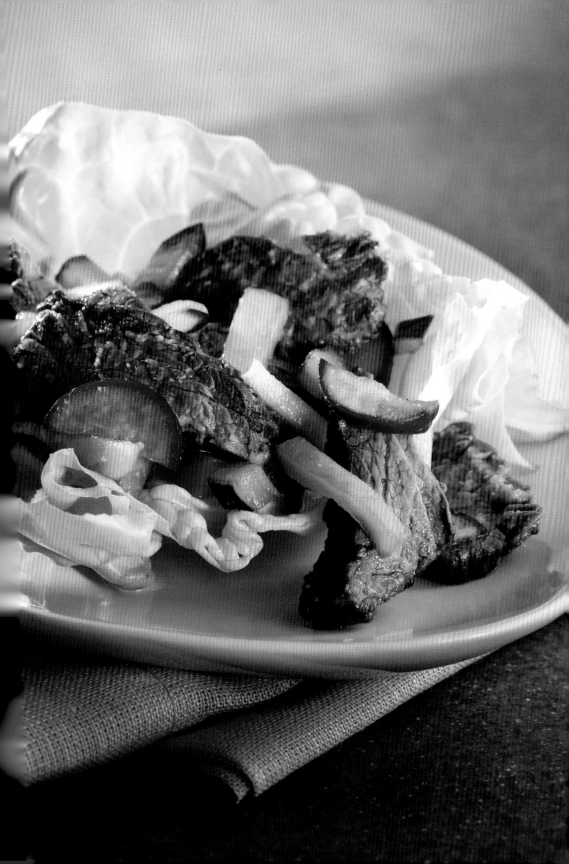

Braised Beef and Cabbage

Using cheaper cuts of beef like chuck or bottom round results in a longer cooking time, but it's all unattended and the resulting fork-tender meat is worth it. Also, you'll be hard-pressed to find a better value vegetable than a head of cabbage, making this a great budget-friendly meal. SERVES 4

1 tablespoon canola oil

½ teaspoon kosher salt, divided

1½ pounds extra-lean beef chuck or bottom round, cut into 1½-inch cubes (see page 138)

1 large head green cabbage, shredded

4 cloves garlic, coarsely chopped

1 cup reduced-sodium beef broth, divided

Grated zest of ½ orange

1 tablespoon low-fat sour cream

Heat the canola oil in a large heavy sauté pan or Dutch oven over medium-high heat. Season the beef with ¼ teaspoon of the salt. Working in batches if needed, sear all sides of the meat, 2 to 3 minutes on each side. As the meat is browned, transfer it to a plate. Still over medium-high heat, add half the cabbage. Sauté, stirring, until wilted, about 2 to 4 minutes. Add the remaining cabbage and repeat. Stir in the garlic, cooking 30 seconds. Add ½ cup of the broth, stirring to get the tasty bits off the bottom of the pan. Add the remaining ½ cup broth and ¼ teaspoon salt, and bring to a boil. Return the meat to the pot, cover with a lid, and reduce the heat to low so the liquid is simmering. Let simmer until the meat is fork tender, about 1½ hours. Taste and adjust the seasonings with salt and pepper as needed. Remove from the heat, and stir in the orange zest and sour cream. Serve.

DO THE DASH Cabbage is a good source of vitamin C, folate, and vitamin K. A recent study found that higher intakes of vitamin K can reduce coronary artery calcification which, in turn, may slash heart disease risk. Don't forget to serve up a side salad with this dish.

SHOPPING TIP To save time, you can also ask the butcher to cube the meat at no extra cost.

NUTRITION Per Serving: 317 calories; 42 grams protein; 15 grams carbohydrate; 6 grams fiber; 10 grams fat (2 grams saturated); 581 mg sodium

Polenta Casserole with Pork Chops

Polenta and pork chops are both inexpensive ingredients that are transformed into a tasty casserole. *Serves 6*

1 pound center-cut boneless pork chops

½ teaspoon salt, divided

¼ teaspoon freshly ground black pepper

½ teaspoon dried thyme

2 teaspoons canola oil

1 cup low-fat ricotta cheese

4 ounces prepared basil pesto

⅓ cup grated Parmigiano-Reggiano cheese

1 large egg, beaten

4 cups skim milk, plus more as needed

1½ cups coarse cornmeal

Preheat the oven to 350°F. Season the pork chops with ¼ teaspoon of the salt and the pepper and thyme. Heat the canola oil in a medium sauté pan or skillet over medium-high heat. Quickly sear the pork chops, just 2 minutes on each side. Remove the pork chops from the pan and reserve. Combine the ricotta cheese, pesto, Parmigiano-Reggiano cheese, and egg in a bowl. Reserve. Coat a 9 x 13-inch rectangular baking dish with cooking spray; set aside. In a medium pot, bring the milk and remaining salt to a simmer over medium-high heat. Lower the heat to medium-low, and pour the cornmeal into the milk, while vigorously whisking. Cook, stirring constantly, until the polenta is thick, 3 to 5 minutes. Remove from the heat.

Pour half of the polenta into the prepared baking dish, using a spatula to spread it in an even layer. Working quickly, spread half of the ricotta mixture on top of the polenta. Add the pork chops, followed by another layer of the remaining ricotta mixture. Top with the remaining polenta. If the polenta has gotten too thick, return to the stove over medium heat, add more milk, and whisk until the polenta is soft again. Bake, uncovered, until the casserole is heated through and the top is lightly golden, about 15 minutes.

DO THE DASH Several studies suggest that higher intakes of the dairy protein whey can aid in controlling blood pressure numbers. It turns out that low-fat ricotta cheese is among the best dairy sources of whey.

SHOPPING TIP If you are concerned about purchasing genetically modified foods, consider splurging for organic cornmeal. Much of the corn grown in the U.S. is now genetically modified. Remember that cornmeal counts toward your whole-grain servings.

NUTRITION Per Serving: 472 calories; 32 grams protein; 35 grams carbohydrate; 2 grams fiber; 22 grams fat (7 grams saturated); 630 mg sodium

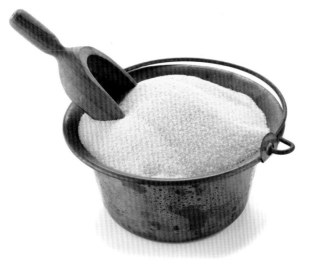

Shepherd's Pie

This lightened-up version of shepherd's pie has pureed cauliflower standing in for the traditional mashed potatoes. *SERVES 6*

1 (1-pound) head cauliflower, chopped

½ cup skim milk

½ kosher salt, divided

2 teaspoons canola oil

1 pound lean ground lamb

2 cloves garlic, minced

½ (16-ounce) bag frozen green peas, thawed

Preheat the oven to 350°F. Bring a large pot of salted water to a boil over high heat. Cook the cauliflower until tender, about 8 minutes, depending on size of the cauliflower florets. Drain the cauliflower in a colander. Puree the cauliflower with the milk and ¼ teaspoon of the salt in a food processor or blender, until smooth. Set aside.

Heat the canola oil in a medium sauté pan or skillet over medium-high heat. Add the lamb and the remaining ¼ teaspoon salt. Sauté, stirring occasionally to break up the meat, until browned, 5 to 7 minutes. Add the garlic and the peas, and cook 2 minutes longer, stirring constantly. Remove from the heat, and drain any remaining oil from the lamb. Transfer the mixture to an ovenproof 9 x 13-inch casserole dish. Spread the cauliflower over the top. Bake, uncovered, until the top is golden and the casserole is hot throughout, 20 to 25 minutes. Serve.

DO THE DASH Cauliflower is chock-full of both vitamin C and vitamin K. Plus, swapping it for mashed potatoes trims about 400 calories from the recipe.

SHOPPING TIP Richly flavored ground lamb can contain fairly high amounts of fat calories, so look for the word "lean" on the label. If you can't find ground lamb, substitute with lean ground beef.

NUTRITION Per Serving: 280 calories; 17 grams protein; 10 grams carbohydrate; 4 grams fiber; 19 grams fat (8 grams saturated); 309 mg sodium

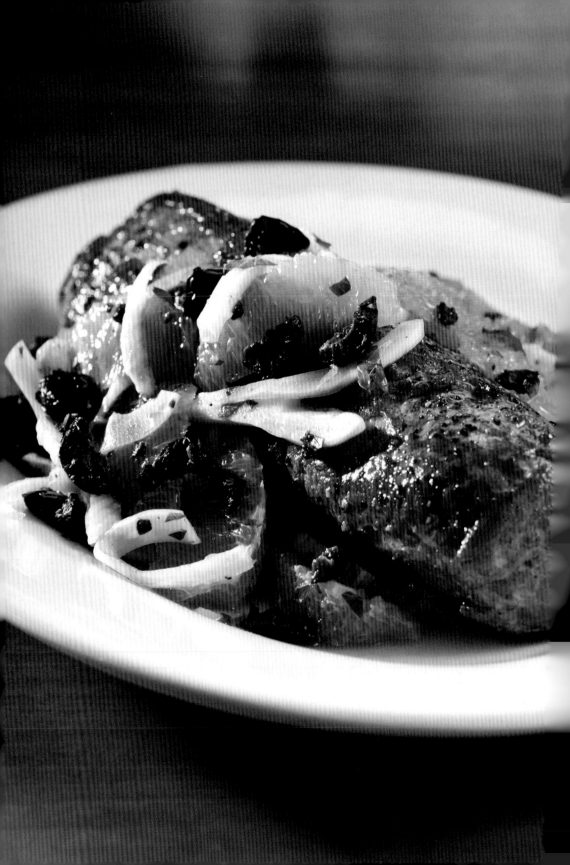

Pork Tenderloin with Orange and Fennel Relish

The trick to cooking pork tenderloin is to remove it from the oven at the correct internal temperature before it overcooks. Also, if you're not comfortable supreming the oranges, just substitute with 2 (11-ounce) cans of drained mandarin oranges. *SERVES 4*

4 oranges

3 large fennel bulbs, trimmed of feathery stalks and chopped

½ cup coarsely chopped parsley

½ cup pitted black olives, coarsely chopped

1½ tablespoons extra-virgin olive oil

½ teaspoon kosher salt, divided

½ teaspoon freshly ground black pepper, divided

1 (1-pound) pork tenderloin

2 teaspoons canola oil

Preheat the oven to 400°F. Make the orange and fennel relish: Supreme the oranges into a bowl (see page 138) . Add the fennel, parsley, and olives. Stir to combine, and drizzle with the olive oil. Season with ¼ teaspoon of the salt and ¼ teaspoon of the pepper and set aside.

Season the pork tenderloin with the remaining ¼ teaspoon salt and remaining ¼ teaspoon pepper. Heat the canola oil in a ovenproof sauté pan or skillet over high heat. Sauté the pork on each side until golden brown, 2 to 3 minutes per side. Roast the pork in the oven until a meat thermometer registers 145°F, about 10 minutes. Remove from the oven and let rest for 10 minutes. Thinly slice the pork diagonally. Serve with the orange and fennel relish.

DO THE DASH Herbs like parsley add bright flavor to dishes such as this one in lieu of lots of salt. Plus, they provide a number of disease-fighting compounds like antioxidants.

SHOPPING TIP Pork tenderloin is nearly as lean as chicken breast, but with more flavor and a less hefty price tag. It should be a more popular cut of meat at the butcher counter.

NUTRITION Per Serving: 324 calories; 27 grams protein; 31 grams carbohydrate; 9 grams fiber; 12 grams fat (2 grams saturated); 552 mg sodium

FISH AND SHELLFISH

Increasingly, research has shown that higher intakes of seafood—particularly those rich in omega-3 fats like salmon and trout—can help us dodge a number of maladies including heart disease. Unfortunately, it can also be one of the more expensive additions to your grocery cart. Never fear—with a few tricks up your sleeve, there are ways to add seafood to your diet and deliciousness to your dinner plate without blowing up your food budget.

First off, you can try cooking with more-affordable fish, like catfish and tilapia. Also, keep an eye out for sales; the fish counter will often have weekly specials. Also, stock up on unseasoned frozen fish and shellfish like salmon and shrimp which are generally high in quality but more budget friendly than fresh options. Another alternative is to buy smaller quantities of the pricey stuff like wild salmon and augment the dish with an abundance of other DASH Diet recommended ingredients, like vegetables and beans. Yet, it's sometimes simply worth splurging and finding other ways to cut down on your food budget.

Mussels with Coconut Milk and Lemongrass

Most of the mussels sold at fish counters these days come de-bearded and fairly clean. Still, mussels should get a quick soak in a bowl of water to make sure they are free of any grit. To use lemongrass, smash it with a large chef's knife, remove the outer layers, and chop the small inner layers, which are full of flavor. *SERVES 4*

1 teaspoon canola oil

1 stalk lemongrass, chopped

2 cloves garlic, minced

1-inch piece fresh ginger, minced

1 jalapeño pepper, seeded and finely chopped

1 cup light coconut milk

2 pounds mussels, scrubbed and de-bearded

2 tablespoons chopped cilantro

1 tablespoon unsalted butter

French bread, sliced (optional)

Heat the canola oil in a large, heavy saucepan over medium-high heat. Add the lemongrass, garlic, ginger, and jalapeño. Cook, stirring constantly, until fragrant, 30 seconds to 1 minute. Add the coconut milk and increase the heat to high. Once the liquid reaches a boil, add the mussels and cover with a lid. Cook until most of the mussels are open, 4 to 5 minutes. Discard any unopened mussels. Transfer the mussels into four large bowls, leaving the broth in the pan. Place the pan over high heat, and add the cilantro and the butter. Boil the broth until reduced and thickened, 2 to 3 minutes, then pour over the mussels. If desired, serve with French bread for dipping.

DO THE DASH Inexpensive mussels are a rich source of a number of vital nutrients including vitamin B12, selenium, zinc, B vitamins, and heart-healthy omega-3 fats. Farm-raised mussels are also considered a sustainable seafood option as they actually clean the water they are being raised in.

SHOPPING TIP When purchasing mussels and other seafood from the grocery store, make it the last item you pick up before hitting the checkout to assure that the product stays fresh. Also, consider putting a cooler in your car to keep the fish cool for the drive home.

NUTRITION Per Serving (without bread): 278 calories; 28 grams protein; 12 grams carbohydrate; 0 gram fiber; 13 grams fat (6 grams saturated); 657 mg sodium

Salmon with Honey Glaze

The packages of frozen salmon in most supermarkets are a few dollars cheaper per pound than the fresh fillets from the fish counter, so that's my choice for this Asian-inspired dish. Pair this with Chinese forbidden rice (also called black rice) and steamed vegetables for a healthy, simple meal. *SERVES 2*

⅓ cup reduced-sodium soy sauce

1 tablespoon mustard

2 teaspoons grated fresh ginger

2 fillets (¾ pound) frozen salmon, thawed

1 teaspoon honey

In a small, shallow bowl, whisk the soy sauce, mustard, and ginger until combined. Pat the salmon fillets dry with paper towels and put in the marinade skin-side down. Cover and refrigerate for 20 minutes. Preheat the broiler. Line a rimmed baking sheet with foil. Remove the salmon from the marinade and pat dry. Place the salmon skin-side down on the prepared baking sheet and drizzle with the honey. Broil 3 to 4 minutes, then rotate the baking sheet, and cook until desired doneness in center, 3 to 4 minutes longer.

DO THE DASH Salmon is one of the leading sources of omega-3 fatty acids in the grocery store. By helping limit inflammation in the body, omega-3s are considered champions for heart health. Studies also suggest that higher blood levels of fish-derived omega-3 fats can help lower blood pressure numbers.

SHOPPING TIP Look for salmon that is labeled "wild," which is almost always a more sustainable choice than farmed salmon, often labeled "Atlantic."

NUTRITION Per Serving: 368 calories; 35 grams protein; 4 grams carbohydrate; 0 gram fiber; 23 grams fat (5 grams saturated); 661 mg sodium

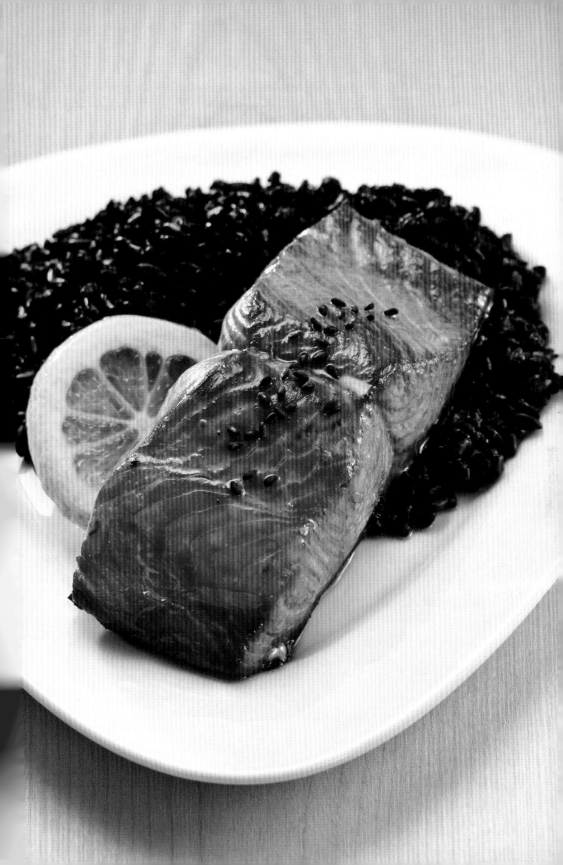

Mojo-Marinated Shrimp Kebabs

Mojo is the name of a Cuban sauce made from sour oranges, but the taste can be replicated with a combination of orange juice and lime juice. Just a dip in a citrus marinade delivers a wallop of flavor to the shrimp. *Serves 4*

Grated zest of 1 orange plus juice of 3 oranges

Grated zest of 1 lime plus juice of 5 limes

3 cloves garlic, minced

1 tablespoon chili powder

1½ teaspoons ground cumin

1 teaspoon dried oregano

1½ pounds medium shrimp, peeled and deveined

2 tablespoons unsalted butter, melted

Grated zest and juice of 1 lemon

2 teaspoons hot sauce

Soak 20 to 25 (6-inch) wooden skewers in water for 30 minutes. Combine the orange juice, orange zest, lime juice, lime zest, garlic, chili powder, cumin, and oregano in a small bowl. Add the shrimp and stir to coat with the marinade. Cover and refrigerate for 30 to 45 minutes. Preheat the broiler. Remove the shrimp from the marinade. Thread skewers with 4 to 5 shrimps each, and place on a rimmed baking sheet. Mix the melted butter with the lemon zest and juice and the hot sauce in a small bowl. Brush the shrimp with the sauce. Broil the shrimp until cooked through and pink, 2 to 3 minutes.

DO THE DASH   Shrimp are considered a lean protein option, with a 3-ounce serving containing only 90 calories. If possible, seek out North American shrimp which are an environmentally more responsible option than imported shrimp from Asia.

SHOPPING TIP   Chili powders can vary greatly with respect to their heat. Some are mild while others are volcano-like, so take a small taste before adding to recipes and adjust the amount appropriately.

NUTRITION   Per Serving: 250 calories; 35 grams protein; 7 grams carbohydrate; 0 grams fiber; 9 grams fat (4 grams saturated); 251 mg sodium

Blackened Catfish Tacos

This classic Cajun dish uses bold seasonings that work well in a taco. Packaged Cajun spice normally contains a mixture of several spices including paprika, garlic, oregano, and cayenne, as well as a good amount of salt. For a DASH-friendly version, see my Low-Sodium Cajun Spice Mix below. *SERVES 4, MAKES 8 TACOS*

2 tablespoons low-fat mayonnaise
1 tablespoon apple cider vinegar
⅓ head large green cabbage, shredded
2 carrots, shredded
1 pound catfish fillets

1 tablespoon Low-Sodium Cajun Spice Mix (see below)
¼ teaspoon freshly ground black pepper
8 (6-inch) whole wheat tortillas

Preheat the oven to 400°F. Line a rimmed baking sheet with foil. Make the slaw: Combine the mayonnaise and vinegar in a medium bowl. Stir in the cabbage and the carrots.

Cut the catfish into 1-inch strips, and season both sides with low-sodium Cajun spice and pepper. Transfer the catfish to the prepared baking sheet. Bake until the catfish is cooked, 10 to 12 minutes. Spread the tortillas on a second baking sheet and warm in the oven while the catfish is cooking. To serve, layer catfish pieces onto each tortilla. Top with slaw and serve.

DO THE DASH   Fish tacos are a perfect way to add a healthy dose of vegetables to mealtime. Here, you could even add shredded zucchini and sliced bell pepper to the mix.

SHOPPING TIP   When selecting tortillas for these tacos, make sure the first ingredient listed on the package is whole wheat, not wheat flour or enriched wheat flour, which are simply code for white flour.

NUTRITION   Per Serving: 353 calories; 23 grams protein; 33 grams carbohydrate; 3 grams fiber; 14 grams fat (3 grams saturated); 393 mg sodium

Low-Sodium Cajun Spice Mix: In a small bowl, combine 1 tablespoon paprika, 2 teaspoons dried thyme, 2 teaspoons cayenne pepper, 1½ teaspoons freshly ground black pepper, 1 teaspoon garlic powder, and 1 teaspoon kosher salt. Yield will be more than needed for recipe. Reserve leftover seasoning for another use.

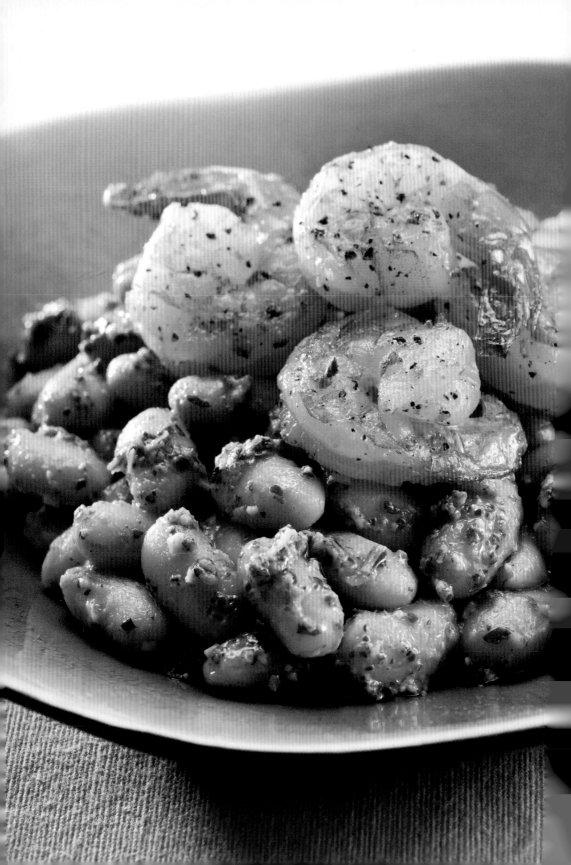

White Beans, Pesto, and Shrimp

Tender cannellini beans have a very neutral flavor, which allows them to add a little heft to this dish without distracting from the flavor of the shrimp and pesto. *SERVES 4*

2 (15.5-ounce) cans cannellini beans, rinsed and drained

⅓ cup prepared pesto

1 tablespoon extra-virgin olive oil

1 pound medium shrimp, peeled and deveined

¼ teaspoon freshly ground black pepper

Juice of 1 lemon

Combine the beans and pesto thoroughly in a large bowl. Heat the olive oil in a large skillet over high heat. Sauté the shrimp until pink, 2 to 3 minutes. Remove from the heat and season with pepper and lemon juice. Divide the pesto beans among serving bowls, top with the shrimp, and serve.

DO THE DASH Cannellini beans are a significant source of dietary fiber, which the DASH Diet encourages people to eat more of as studies suggest it reduces one's risk for heart disease, certain cancers and obesity. Look for Eden Organic brand of canned beans, as they offer "no salt added" options.

SHOPPING TIP Store-bought pesto can be very high in sodium, so compare labels for the lowest-salt options, or, better yet, pull out the food processor and make your own. The Web is chockablock with simple, creative pesto recipes.

NUTRITION Per Serving: 392 calories; 32 grams protein; 33 grams carbohydrate; 12 grams fiber; 14 grams fat (3 grams saturated); 416 mg sodium

Whole Trout with Garlic and Lemon

Whole trout looks intimidating. But when you buy it, most of the time (ask!), it's already been split in half. All you have to do is stuff it with deliciousness like herbs and lemon, and place it in the oven. Get ready to be impressed. *Serves 4*

3 tablespoons unsalted butter, cut into pieces, at room temperature

⅓ cup chopped parsley

Grated zest and juice of 1 lemon

Kosher salt and freshly ground black pepper

2 medium cloves garlic

1 whole lemon, sliced

4 (¾-pound) whole trout

1½ tablespoons olive oil

Preheat the oven to 350°F. Combine the butter, parsley, lemon zest, lemon juice, and ½ teaspoon of the pepper in a small bowl. Mince the garlic very fine, and then mix into the butter mixture with a spoon. Line a rimmed baking sheet with foil and coat with cooking spray. Open each trout, and season with the salt and remaining ¼ teaspoon pepper. Stuff each trout with one-fourth of the butter mixture and 1 or 2 slices of lemon, and place on the prepared baking sheet. Drizzle the olive oil over the fish. Bake the trout until their flesh is flaky, about 30 minutes. Remove from the oven, and serve.

DO THE DASH Similar to salmon, rainbow trout is an excellent source of heart-friendly omega-3 fats. Much of what is available at stores is farmed, but environmental groups consider inland trout farming to be a sustainable, non-polluting practice.

SHOPPING TIP Cooking fish whole results in a more memorable dish since the skin and bones contribute to flavor. Most fish counters sell whole trout that has already been cleaned.

NUTRITION Per Serving: 371 calories; 36 grams protein; 5 grams carbohydrate; 1 gram fiber; 23 grams fat (9 grams saturated); 353 mg sodium

Tuna-Stuffed Red Bell Peppers

Stuffing red bell peppers with tuna salad creates a light, no-cook meal option. Try serving with some whole grains like quinoa or brown rice. Find roasted red bell peppers either in the olive bar or the prepared food aisle at most supermarkets. *SERVES 4*

3 tablespoons low-fat mayonnaise

2 teaspoons freshly squeezed lemon juice

¼ teaspoon kosher salt

¼ teaspoon freshly ground black pepper

2 tablespoons chopped pitted green olives

2 (6-ounce) cans albacore tuna in spring water, drained

2 stalks celery, chopped

1 carrot, grated

1 cucumber, peeled and chopped

4 whole roasted red bell peppers

In a large bowl, combine the mayonnaise, lemon juice, salt, pepper, and olives. Add the tuna, celery, carrot, and cucumber. Use a fork to combine the tuna with the vegetables. Taste and adjust the seasonings as needed. Cut each of the peppers down the center, then fill equally with the tuna salad.

DO THE DASH Eating plenty of water-rich foods like celery and cucumber can help keep you hydrated. When you do not consume adequate water the body will compensate by retaining sodium, which could raise blood pressure numbers.

SHOPPING TIP If your food budget permits, purchase canned albacore tuna from smaller companies like Wild Planet. Their products have a higher level of disease-fighting omega-3s because the tuna is cooked in the can rather than before packing, so less is lost in the process. In addition, they generally catch smaller tuna, which hasn't had as much time to accumulate toxins like mercury.

NUTRITION Per Serving: 204 calories; 22 grams protein; 12 grams carbohydrate; 4 grams fiber; 7 grams fat (1 gram saturated); 332 mg sodium

VEGETARIAN

Even hardened carnivores should embrace one or more meat-free meals a week. Studies suggest that even part-time vegetarians (aka flexitarians) experience health benefits such as reduced heart disease and trimmer waistlines. Plus, the DASH Diet encourages the increased consumption of plant-based foods as they are often chock-full of nutrients shown to have blood pressure–lowering benefits. There are plenty of ways to get the protein you need without eating meat, and you'll feel good about your choice for health, environmental, and ethical reasons. Embracing Meatless Monday's is also a cheaper route to go. Vegetarian sources of protein like quinoa, edamame, and tofu are much cheaper than their meat counterparts.

Pitas with Baked Falafel and Cucumber-Yogurt Sauce

Baking the falafel makes them a lot healthier than the traditional fried variety. With the delicious sauce, you'll barely notice the taste difference. *SERVES 4, MAKES 8 PITA HALF SANDWICHES*

For the falafel:

2 (15-ounce) cans chickpeas, rinsed and drained

2 cloves garlic, minced

Juice of ½ lemon

3 tablespoons flour

½ teaspoon baking powder

¼ teaspoon kosher salt

1 teaspoon ground coriander

½ teaspoon red pepper flakes

1 large egg

For the cucumber-yogurt sauce:

1 garlic clove

1 cup nonfat Greek yogurt

1 tablespoon freshly squeezed lemon juice

2 tablespoons finely diced cucumber

¼ teaspoon kosher salt

To serve:

4 small whole-wheat pita breads, sliced in half

2 medium carrots, grated

1 large tomato, sliced

Make the falafel: Preheat the oven to 425°F. Line a rimmed baking sheet with foil and coat with cooking spray. Add the chickpeas, garlic, lemon juice, flour, baking powder, salt, coriander, pepper flakes, and egg to a food processor. Process 30 seconds to 1 minute until somewhat pureed but still chunky. Form the falafel mixture into balls about the size of a golf ball, placing on the prepared baking sheet. Bake until slightly crisped on the outside, about 30 minutes. Meanwhile, make the cucumber-yogurt sauce: Mince the garlic, then use the side of the knife to make a paste of the garlic. Combine the garlic, yogurt, lemon juice, cucumber, and salt in a small bowl. Taste and adjust the seasonings as needed.

To serve, place falafels in the pita pockets. Garnish with the sauce, shredded carrots, and tomato slices.

DO THE DASH Chickpeas are a leading source of dietary fiber, which aids in shedding excess pounds. If you need to lose weight, even a small amount of weight loss will help to lower risks of developing high blood pressure and other serious health conditions. Make sure to give canned chickpeas a good rinse to rid much of the excess sodium.

SHOPPING TIP   Like all bread products, look for pitas with a whole grain as the first ingredient, such as whole wheat flour. To control calories, choose smaller-size pitas.

NUTRITION   Per Serving: 423 calories; 22 grams protein; 76 grams carbohydrate; 13 grams fiber; 5 grams fat (1 gram saturated); 509 mg sodium

Black Bean Burgers

These healthy black bean burgers will even appease a hardened carnivore. Also, feel free to play around with the recipe, substituting different grains, nuts, beans, and toppings. *Serves 4*

1¼ cups canned black beans, rinsed and drained

1 cup cooked brown rice

¾ cup unsalted cashews

1 tablespoon reduced-sodium soy sauce

¼ cup parsley sprigs

1 large egg

¼ teaspoon kosher salt

¼ teaspoon freshly ground black pepper

2 tablespoons canola oil

4 whole-wheat hamburger buns

1 tomato, sliced

1 cup packed baby spinach

Add the black beans, brown rice, cashews, soy sauce, parsley, egg, salt, and pepper to a food processor. Pulse the mixture until smooth, about 1 minute. Form into 4 patties. Heat the canola oil in a medium nonstick sauté pan or skillet over medium-high heat. Carefully add the patties (they are fragile), and cook until slightly browned, 2 to 3 minutes on each side. Serve on the buns with tomatoes, spinach, and any desired condiments.

DO THE DASH   The creators of the DASH Diet stress the importance of eating plenty of antioxidant-rich foods. It turns out that black beans have an antioxidant capacity on par with fruits and vegetables.

SHOPPING TIP   Some grocery stores now sell cooked brown rice in the freezer department to help slash prep time.

NUTRITION   Per Serving: 438 calories; 15 grams protein; 47 grams carbohydrate; 8 grams fiber; 23 grams fat (4 grams saturated); 406 mg sodium

Scallion Quinoa with Corn and Squash

Quinoa is a grain-like seed crop native to the Andes. It's a complete protein source and a good source of fiber, so it's a much healthier alternative to pasta salads for potlucks and cookouts. Serve this versatile dish at any temperature and feel free to use other vegetables as you like. *Serves 6*

1½ cups quinoa

3 cups water

1½ cups nonfat Greek yogurt

3 scallions, green parts only, coarsely chopped

1½ tablespoons reduced-sodium soy sauce

1 tablespoon unsalted butter

2 yellow squash, finely diced

2 cups fresh or frozen corn kernels (about 4 ears corn)

1 cup chopped bok choy

4 ounces soft goat cheese, crumbled

Add the quinoa and water to a medium pot. Bring to a boil over high heat, cover, reduce the heat to low, and simmer until tender and the water has been absorbed, about 15 minutes. Remove from the heat. Meanwhile, puree the yogurt, scallions, and soy sauce in a food processor or blender until smooth, about 1 minute. Reserve. Melt the butter in a sauté pan or skillet over medium-high heat. Add the squash, and sauté 2 to 3 minutes. Add the corn and the bok choy and sauté, stirring, until the bok choy is wilted, 2 to 3 minutes longer. Transfer the quinoa to a large serving bowl. Add the yogurt mixture and stir to combine. Then add the vegetables and mix. Top with the cheese and serve.

DO THE DASH   The DASH Diet recommends emphasizing whole grains, and there is no better place to start than quinoa, laced with many vital nutrients including impressive amounts of magnesium, which has been shown to help improve blood sugar numbers. Plus, it cooks up in half the time of brown rice.

SHOPPING TIP   An increasing number of larger grocery stores now carry quinoa. Look for it in the bulk bin section or packaged in the health food section.

NUTRITION   Per Serving: 285 calories; 15 grams protein; 38 grams carbohydrate; 5 grams fiber; 9 grams fat (4 grams saturated); 221 mg sodium

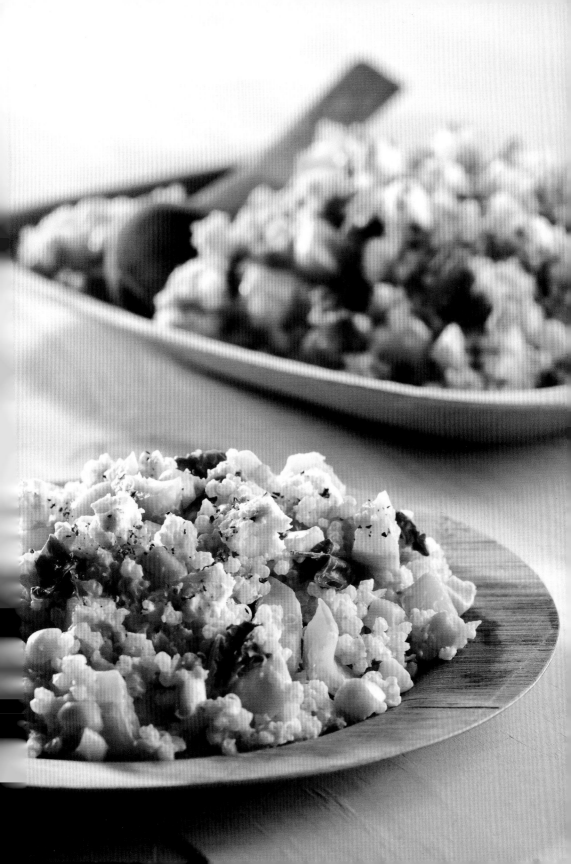

Oven-Baked Hash Browns with Eggs

I'll be honest—these oven-baked hash browns aren't as pretty as their fried counterpart, but they're just as tasty and a heck of a lot healthier. Served with fried eggs, hash browns are turned into a meal. *SERVES 4*

4 medium to large russet potatoes (1½ to 2 pounds), peeled

2 teaspoons freshly squeezed lemon juice

½ teaspoon kosher salt

½ teaspoon freshly ground black pepper

2½ tablespoons olive oil, divided

4 large eggs

Preheat the oven to 400°F. Line a rimmed baking sheet with foil. Put a grater in a large bowl, and shred the potatoes. Using 1 or 2 paper towels, blot the excess moisture from the potatoes. Add the lemon juice, salt, and pepper, and stir to combine. Using a tablespoon measurer, drop small mounds of potatoes onto the prepared baking sheet, flattening each one. Drizzle the potatoes with 2 tablespoons of the olive oil. Bake until crisped around the edges, 40 to 50 minutes. Meanwhile, in a large nonstick skillet, heat ½ tablespoon olive oil over medium-high heat. Crack the eggs into the pan, and cook until the egg whites set, 1 to 2 minutes. Flip the eggs, and cook the yolks just briefly, about 30 seconds to 1 minute. Remove from the heat. To serve, divide the hash browns among serving plates and top each with an egg.

DO THE DASH   Not just for breakfast, eggs are an inexpensive source of a range of nutrients including vitamin D, vitamin B12, selenium, and riboflavin, a B vitamin that could offer blood pressure benefits according to a recent *American Journal of Clinical Nutrition* study.

SHOPPING TIP   When using olive oil for cooking purposes, consider choosing light versions, which have a more neutral flavor and higher smoke point than extra-virgin. Save extra-virgin olive oil for salads, dips, and other non-heat applications.

NUTRITION   Per Serving: 297 calories; 10 grams protein; 35 grams carbohydrate; 4 grams fiber; 14 grams fat (3 grams saturated); 374 mg sodium

Rosemary Focaccia with Roasted Tomatoes

Made from whole wheat pizza dough, this focaccia is a healthier twist on the classic. Sun-dried tomatoes packed in olive oil can be substituted for the fresh tomatoes. *SERVES 4*

Flour, as needed

1 ball (about 8 ounces) whole wheat pizza dough, at room temperature

2 tablespoons olive oil, divided

Leaves of 3 sprigs rosemary

¼ teaspoon kosher salt

1 small red onion, sliced

⅓ pound tomatoes, sliced (about ⅔ cup)

⅓ pound jarred or frozen artichoke hearts, sliced (about ⅔ cup)

Preheat the oven to 425°F. Sprinkle 1 to 2 tablespoons flour onto a work surface. Place the pizza dough on the work surface and gently knead and stretch the dough. Drizzle an 8 x 12-inch glass baking dish with 1 tablespoon of the olive oil and spread the pizza dough in the dish, pressing the dough down into the bottom of the dish. Use your fingers to punch tiny indentations into the top of the dough. Press the rosemary leaves into the dough, and sprinkle with salt. Layer the onion, tomatoes, and artichokes on the dough. Bake until the focaccia is puffy and golden, 25 to 30 minutes. Drizzle with the remaining 1 tablespoon olive oil and cut into pieces.

DO THE DASH In a recent U.K. study, people who consumed three servings of whole grains a day, such as whole wheat pizza dough, for three months lowered their systolic blood pressure by 5 to 6 millimeters of mercury—which slashed their risks for heart disease and stroke by 15 and 25 percent, respectively.

SHOPPING TIP Some supermarkets sell balls of whole wheat pizza dough in the refrigerator section. You can also try your local pizzeria, which should be more than happy to sell you their premade dough for a few bucks.

NUTRITION Per Serving: 214 calories; 6 grams protein; 32 grams carbohydrate; 4 grams fiber; 9 grams fat (1 gram saturated); 408 mg sodium

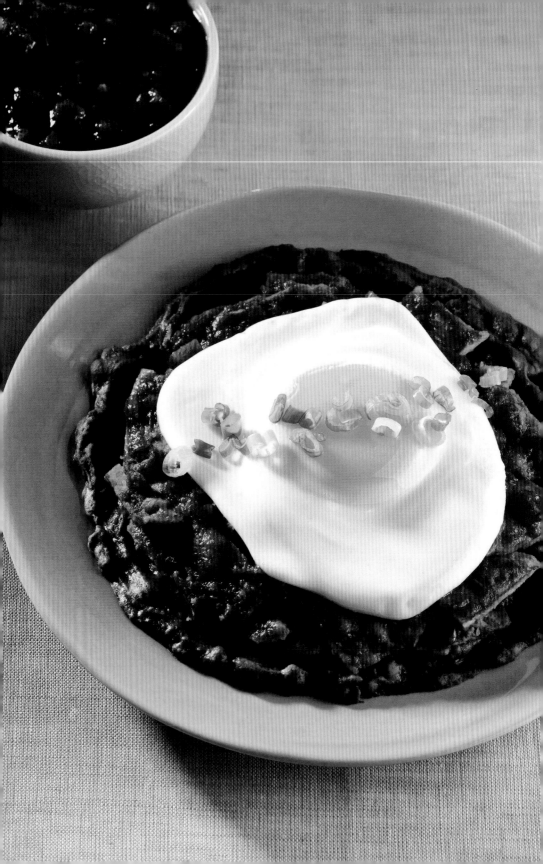

Chilaquiles

This spin on a traditional Mexican dish can be eaten any time of day. The tortilla chips soak up all the flavor of the salsa, making this superfast dish taste like it was slow-cooked. *Serves 4*

1 cup salsa

1 (9-ounce bag) baked tortilla chips, slightly broken

1 (15-ounce) can refried black beans

4 large eggs

2 scallions, chopped

Heat the salsa and chips in a large nonstick skillet over medium-high heat. Cook, stirring often, until the chips are soft from absorbing the sauce, 3 to 4 minutes. Meanwhile, spread the refried beans in a microwave-safe dish and heat in the microwave until hot, 3 to 4 minutes. Divide the beans among four plates and layer the chips on top, adding any salsa not absorbed. Wipe out the pan, coat with cooking spray, and heat over medium-high heat. Crack the eggs into the pan, and cook until the egg whites are set, 1 to 2 minutes. Flip the eggs and cook the yolks just briefly, 30 seconds to 1 minute. Remove from the heat. Top each plate with an egg and garnish with scallions. Serve at once.

DO THE DASH If available, try blue corn tortilla chips for this recipe. Made from heirloom blue corn, they have higher antioxidant levels than yellow corn tortilla chips.

SHOPPING TIP Sodium levels can vary greatly for store-bought salsa, tortilla chips, and refried beans, so make sure to read nutrition labels. There are now some no-salt-added tortilla chip options on the market. Also, make sure to purchase canned refried beans with no fat added.

NUTRITION Per Serving: 291 calories; 13 grams protein; 47 grams carbohydrate; 6 grams fiber; 6 grams fat (1 gram saturated); 519 mg sodium

Twice-Baked Sweet Potatoes

Twice-baked potatoes are always a crowd-pleaser. A little honey helps highlight these creamy and delicious sweet potatoes. *SERVES 4*

4 medium sweet potatoes

1½ tablespoons unsalted butter

2 tablespoons reduced-sodium soy sauce

1 tablespoon honey

2 tablespoons heavy cream

2 teaspoons Sriracha, or similar hot sauce

Preheat the oven to 425°F. Line a rimmed baking sheet with foil. Using a fork, poke holes in the sweet potatoes and place on the prepared baking sheet. Bake until a knife can be easily inserted into a potato, about 1 hour. Remove from the oven and let rest until cool enough to handle, 10 to 15 minutes. Increase the oven temperature to 450°F. Cut each sweet potato in half lengthwise, and scoop the flesh into a bowl. Add the butter, soy sauce, honey, cream, and hot sauce, and stir to combine. Spoon the sweet potato mixture into the skins. Return to the baking sheet and bake until hot, 10 to 15 minutes.

DO THE DASH   The orange spuds are chock-full of blood pressure–lowering potassium and beta-carotene. In the body, beta-carotene can be converted to vitamin A to help improve bone, eye, and immune health.

SHOPPING TIP   If you don't have heavy cream on hand or want to use a lighter alternative, you can try using plain 2 percent Greek yogurt.

NUTRITION   Per Serving: 196 calories; 3 grams protein; 31 grams carbohydrate; 4 grams fiber; 7 grams fat (4 grams saturated); 342 mg sodium

Mushroom and Spinach Quesadillas

Mushrooms are an excellent "meaty" low-calorie alternative to meat when making dishes such as quesadillas, burritos, chili and stir-fries. They should be a big part of every diet geared toward weight loss. *SERVES 4*

2 tablespoons canola oil, divided, plus more as needed

1 (10-ounce) container white mushrooms, sliced

1 (9-ounce) bag spinach

2 tomatoes, chopped

2 scallions, chopped

1½ cups shredded low-fat cheddar cheese

4 (10-inch) whole wheat tortilla wraps

Preheat the oven to 300°F. Heat 1 tablespoon of the canola oil in a large sauté pan or skillet over medium-high heat. Add the mushrooms and sauté, stirring occasionally, until the mushrooms are soft, about 10 minutes. Add the spinach and cook, stirring constantly, until wilted, 2 to 3 minutes. Add the tomatoes and scallions, and cook 1 to 2 minutes. Transfer the vegetables to a bowl.

Spread an equal amount of cheese over each tortilla, covering it entirely. Divide the vegetables evenly, spreading on one-half of each tortilla, and fold the other half of the tortilla over the vegetables. Heat the remaining 1 tablespoon canola oil in a medium nonstick skillet over medium-high heat. Add 1 quesadilla, cooking until each side is golden, about 3 minutes per side. Transfer to a rimmed baking sheet, and place in the oven to keep warm. Repeat with the remaining quesadillas, adding more oil as needed. Cut each quesadilla into four pieces, and serve.

SHOPPING TIP   Cheddar cheese is notoriously one of the fattier items in the cheese aisle, so select reduced-fat versions when possible.

NUTRITION   Per Serving: 279 calories; 22 grams protein; 26 grams carbohydrate; 6 grams fiber; 14 grams fat (3 grams saturated); 607 mg sodium

Flatbread with Carrot Puree and Marinated Goat Cheese

Here's proof that you can do a lot of great things with a ball of pizza dough. The goat cheese adds creamy tang, but the real star here is the carrot puree. Eating this dish will be a startling reminder of just how flavorful simple carrots can be. *SERVES 2*

2 teaspoons canola oil

1 cup chopped yellow onion

1 pound carrots, chopped (about 8 to 10)

1 to 1½ cups water

¼ teaspoon kosher salt

¼ teaspoon freshly ground black pepper

1 tablespoon unsalted butter

Flour, as needed

1 ball (about 8 ounces) whole wheat pizza dough, at room temperature

4 ounces soft goat cheese, crumbled

Position a rack in the middle of the oven and preheat the oven to 450°F. Heat the canola oil in a large sauté pan or skillet over medium-high heat. Add the onion and cook until translucent, 2 to 3 minutes. Add the carrots and 1 cup water. Cook until the carrots are tender, about 10 minutes. If the water has evaporated, add the remaining ½ cup water. Remove from the heat and season with salt and pepper. Transfer the carrots to a food processor, add the butter, and puree until smooth, 1 to 2 minutes. Taste and adjust the seasoning as needed.

Dust a work surface and your hands with 1 to 2 tablespoons flour. Remove the pizza dough from its package. Slowly stretch the dough on the back of your knuckles, rotating the dough and stretching it into a circular shape. When the dough is stretched to about 1 foot in diameter, place on the work surface and stretch the dough even more using your fingertips.

Place the dough directly onto the middle rack of the oven. Bake until the crust bottom is browned, about 4 minutes. Using tongs, remove from the oven, and place on the work surface with the bottom of the crust facing up. Spread the carrot puree over the flatbread. Scatter the goat cheese over the puree. Place the flatbread in the oven, again directly on the wire rack. Bake until the crust is browned and the cheese is melted, 4 to 6 minutes longer. Using tongs, carefully remove the flatbread and transfer to the work surface. Cut into pieces and serve.

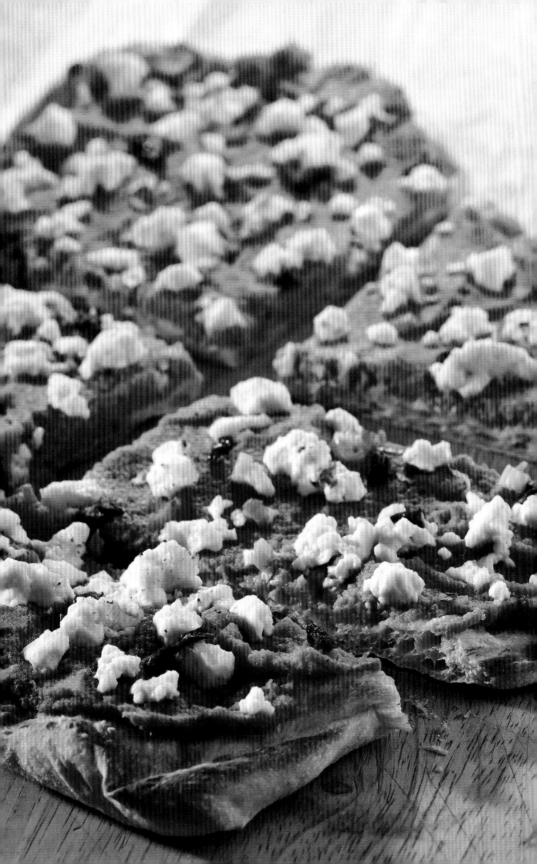

DO THE DASH Bugs Bunny should have been a nutritionist. After all, packed with fiber, potassium, vitamin K, and beta-carotene, his crunchy edible of choice is a nutritional winner.

SHOPPING TIP The DASH Diet certainly does not forbid indulging in a little cheese here and there. When shopping for cheese, consider the horned variety. Goat cheese has about 30 percent less fat than cheddar or Swiss and studies suggest goat milk is richer in omega-3 fats and bone-building calcium than cow's milk is. The protein in goat cheese is also easier to digest.

NUTRITION Per Serving: 300 calories; 11 grams protein; 38 grams carbohydrate; 6 grams fiber; 13 grams fat (6 grams saturated); 563 mg sodium

Broccoli, Sugar Snap Pea, and Edamame Stir-Fry

A veggie extravaganza like stir-fry is always a good idea for a healthy meal when you need to put dinner on the table fast. This one includes edamame for a little boost of protein. *SERVES 4*

1 tablespoon canola oil

2½ cups broccoli florets

1¼ cups frozen shelled edamame, thawed

1½ cups sugar snap peas

2 tablespoons reduced-sodium soy sauce

1 tablespoon grated fresh ginger

2 cloves garlic, minced

½ cup unsalted cashews, coarsely chopped

2 cups cooked brown rice

Heat the canola oil in a medium sized sauté pan or skillet over medium-high heat. Add the broccoli, and sauté, stirring occasionally, until slightly soft, 6 to 8 minutes. Add the edamame and sugar snap peas, and sauté just 1 to 2 minutes. Add the soy sauce, ginger, garlic, and cashews, and sauté, stirring constantly, just 1 to 2 minutes longer. Remove from the heat, and serve with the rice.

DO THE DASH A recent investigation discovered that the daily consumption of foods containing soy isoflavones, such as edamame, can lead to significant drops in blood pressure numbers. Edamame are simply young, green soybeans.

SHOPPING TIP Bags of shelled edamame are in the freezer section alongside other frozen vegetables and legumes. Also, look for frozen brown rice to make this meal an even speedier affair.

NUTRITION Per Serving: 325 calories; 13 grams protein; 38 grams carbohydrate; 6 grams fiber; 15 grams fat (2 grams saturated); 290 mg sodium

DESSERTS

Dessert can be a source of internal conflict—something sweet is called for but brings the associated guilt that comes with the consumption of all that sugar and fat. But, with a few smart substitutions such as whole wheat flour for all-purpose flour there are ways to enjoy a sweet treat that's not entirely unhealthy. Focusing on fruit for dessert is essential because it is packed with both vitamins and natural sugars. This is why most of the desserts in this cookbook are fruit based, like the fruit smoothie and the no-fuss banana raspberry ice cream. If you need a chocolate fix, try the chocolate pudding, where tofu stands in for dairy, making it—dare I say it—guilt-free. These recipes provide ways to satisfy a sweet tooth without unraveling your diet in the process.

Two-Ingredient Banana-Raspberry Ice Cream

Not possible, you say, to make ice cream without an ice cream maker and with just two ingredients? Welcome to the wonder that is the banana which can be frozen and whirled in a food processor to create a consistency similar to ice cream without all the fatty calories. If you prefer, substitute natural peanut butter for the raspberry preserves.   *SERVES 2*

3 to 4 ripe bananas, cut into 1-inch pieces

2 tablespoons raspberry preserves

Place the bananas in a shallow container, and leave in the freezer until frozen, about 2 hours minimum. Transfer to a food processor and add the preserves. Puree until smooth and the consistency of ice cream, 1 to 2 minutes. Serve at once.

DO THE DASH   The rumors are true: Bananas are a leading source of blood pressure–lowering potassium.

SHOPPING TIP   If possible, look for a preserve which lists raspberries before sugar in the ingredient list and contains no high fructose corn syrup.

NUTRITION   Per Serving: 228 calories; 2 grams protein; 53 grams carbohydrate; 5 gram fiber; 1 gram fat (0 grams saturated); 2 mg sodium

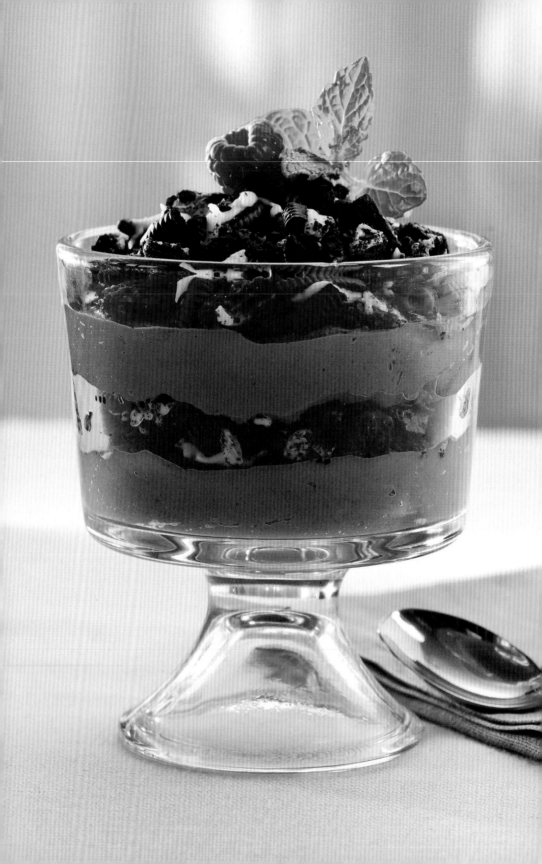

Tofu Chocolate Pudding

This luscious chocolate pudding is so addictively good that you won't believe that it's made with tofu and not cream. Consider garnishing with raspberries. For a real splurge, make a parfait, alternating layers of chocolate pudding and chopped chocolate cookies.   *SERVES 4*

1½ cups dark chocolate chips

1 (14-ounce) package silken tofu, drained

¼ teaspoon salt

2 teaspoons pure vanilla extract

In a microwave-safe dish, melt the chocolate chips in 45-second increments, stirring at each break, until the chocolate is fully melted, 2 to 3 minutes. Puree the chocolate, tofu, salt, and vanilla in a food processor until smooth, just 30 seconds to 1 minute. Transfer the pudding to a container, and refrigerate for 2 hours to set.

DO THE DASH   Dark chocolate contains antioxidants that have been shown to have blood pressure–lowering efficacy.

SHOPPING TIP   You can find silken (soft) tofu alongside the firm tofu, most often in the produce department.

NUTRITION   Per Serving (without cookies): 184 calories; 6 grams protein; 15 grams carbohydrate; 2 grams fiber; 11 grams fat (5 grams saturated);152 mg sodium

Broiled Plums with Vanilla Ice Cream

Broiling the plums enhances their natural sweetness. A fruit sorbet can be substituted for the vanilla ice cream, if desired. *SERVES 4*

2½ teaspoons sugar	8 ripe plums, halved and pitted
1½ teaspoons ground cardamom	½ cup all-natural vanilla ice cream

Preheat the broiler and line a rimmed baking sheet with foil. Combine the sugar and the cardamom in a small bowl. Add the plum halves to the prepared baking sheet, cut-side up, and sprinkle with the sugar mixture. Broil until the edges are slightly charred, 6 to 8 minutes. Let the plums cool slightly. Scoop little balls of ice cream into the center of each cooled plum and serve.

DO THE DASH Step aside more expensive blueberries: A study from Texas Agri Life Research found that, ounce for ounce, plums contain the same amount of age-avenging antioxidants. The darker the plum, the higher the antioxidant payload.

SHOPPING TIP Fat and calorie counts can vary greatly with ice-cream. Look for one with less than 150 calories and 8 grams of fat per ½ cup serving.

NUTRITION Per Serving: 105 calories; 2 grams protein; 21 grams carbohydrate; 2 grams fiber; 2 grams fat (1 gram saturated); 13 mg sodium

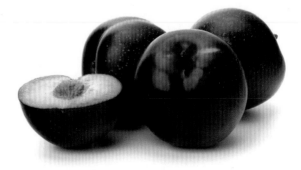

Pineapple Pops

Refreshing Popsicles were always a favorite treat of mine as a child. Making homemade ice pops is very easy and results in healthier and tastier treats than the manufactured kind. If you don't feel like pineapple, substitute any other fruit of choice.   *MAKES 6 POPS*

4 cups chopped fresh pineapple

2 tablespoons sugar, plus more as needed

1 cup water

1½ tablespoons freshly squeezed lime juice, plus more as needed

Pulse the pineapple, sugar, water, and lime juice in a food processor until pureed, about 15 one-second pulses. Adjust the flavor with additional lime juice and sugar as needed. Fill 6 ice pop molds according to the manufacturer's directions and freeze at least overnight. Run the pops under warm water to remove. Serve immediately.

DO THE DASH   Pineapple is a source of vitamin C and manganese, a trace mineral necessary for bone health and blood sugar regulation.

SHOPPING TIP   Buying a whole pineapple and cutting it yourself is almost always much cheaper than purchasing peeled and pre-chopped fruit.

NUTRITION   Per Serving: 72 calories; 1 gram protein; 19 grams carbohydrate; 2 grams fiber; 0 grams fat (0 grams saturated); 1 mg sodium

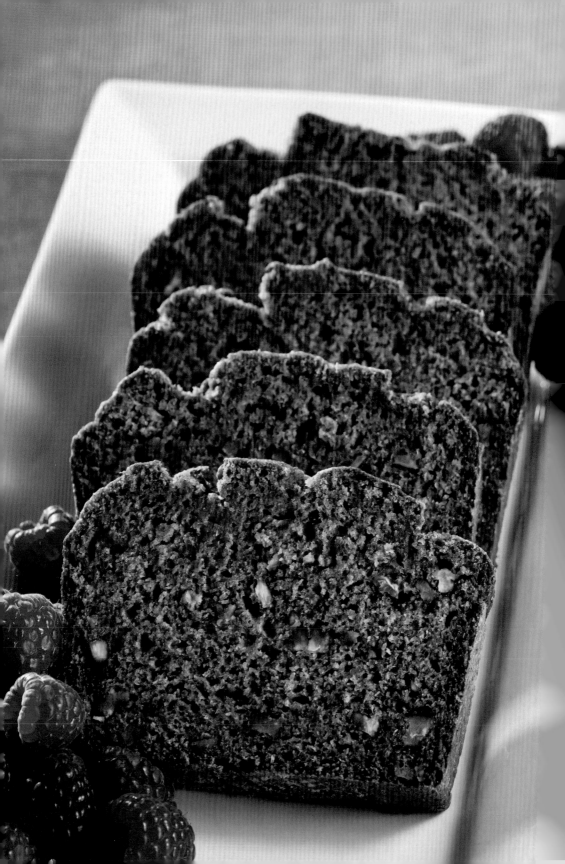

Banana Bread

The magic of this banana bread is that robust tasting maple syrup replaces the sugar in the recipe. Try to use bananas that are very ripe. If using extra ripe bananas, one trick is to puree them in the food processor to make a banana paste. *SERVES 6*

3 ripe bananas

2 tablespoons unsalted butter, melted

1 large egg

½ cup low-fat buttermilk

⅓ cup maple syrup

1 teaspoon vanilla extract

Pinch of salt

1½ teaspoons baking soda

1¼ cups whole wheat flour

½ cup coarsely chopped walnuts (optional)

Preheat the oven to 325°F. Coat an 8 x 4-inch loaf pan with cooking spray. Add the bananas to a large bowl, and use a fork to mash the bananas into a paste-like consistency. Add the butter, egg, buttermilk, and vanilla; stir to combine. Sprinkle the salt and the baking soda over the mixture, and stir to combine. Add the flour, and use a wooden spoon to combine with the other ingredients. Stir in the walnuts, if using. Pour the batter into the prepared loaf pan. Bake until a toothpick inserted into the center of the bread comes out clean, 50 minutes to 1 hour. Slice and serve.

DO THE DASH   When making baked goods, swap out white flour for its whole-grain counterpart more often to boost nutrient and fiber intake. This will help you fulfill the DASH Diet recommended daily whole-grain intake.

SHOPPING TIP   Look for whole wheat pastry flour in the baking aisle as it produces less-dense baked items compared to regular whole wheat flour.

NUTRITION   Per Serving (without nuts): 208 calories; 7 grams protein; 36 grams carbohydrate; 5 grams fiber; 6 grams fat (3 grams saturated); 74 mg sodium

Poached Pears with Lemon Yogurt

Lemon-scented Greek yogurt adds just a touch of tangy richness to these poached pears without a significant amount of calories. *SERVES 4*

4 large pears

2 cups water

⅓ cup sugar

1½ cups freshly squeezed orange juice

1 tablespoon vanilla extract

2 teaspoons ground ginger

1 teaspoon ground cinnamon

¼ cup low-fat plain Greek yogurt

Grated zest of ½ lemon

Peel and core the pears, then trim the bottoms slightly so they sit flat. Add the water, sugar, orange juice, vanilla, ginger, and cinnamon to a large, heavy pot. Bring to a boil and stir to combine the ingredients. Add the pears to the liquid, cover the pan with a lid, and reduce the heat to low. Simmer the pears until tender, about 30 minutes. Remove from the heat, and let the pears cool in the syrup before removing. In a small bowl, combine the yogurt and the lemon zest. To serve, stand each cooled pear upright and spoon an equal amount of the lemon yogurt over the top.

DO THE DASH   Pears are a stellar source of dietary fiber, which makes desserts such as these seem especially filling and satisfying.

SHOPPING TIP   When purchasing vanilla extract, make sure to select only pure ones with no artificial flavorings. The taste different most definitely makes it a worthwhile splurge.

NUTRITION   Per Serving: 222 calories; 3 grams protein; 54 grams carbohydrate; 6 grams fiber; 1 gram fat (0 grams saturated); 9 mg sodium

Forbidden Rice with Mangoes

Chinese black rice, more exotically called "forbidden rice," is one of my favorite purchases at the health food store. It's nutty and delicious—and better yet, so nutritious due to its whole-grain status. Mixed with coconut milk and serve with mangoes, it makes a stellar dessert. *Serves 4*

1 cup forbidden black rice

1¾ cups water

2 tablespoons sugar

Pinch of salt

½ cup light coconut milk

3 mangoes, sliced (see page 137)

¼ cup unsweetened dried coconut

Add the rice, water, sugar, and salt to a medium, heavy pot. Bring to a boil over high heat, cover with a lid, and reduce the heat to low. Simmer until the water is absorbed, 30 to 35 minutes. Add the coconut milk, and let the rice sit for 10 minutes. Stir to combine. To serve, scoop the rice into bowls, and garnish with the mango and coconut.

DO THE DASH Studies suggest that black rice contains the same age-avenging antioxidants as dark-colored fruits like blueberries. If you already follow a healthy, whole-food diet almost all of the time, you can go ahead and indulge by using richer tasting full-fat coconut milk.

SHOPPING TIP If possible, use Altaufo (manila) mangoes, which have a stringless flesh that melts in your mouth.

NUTRITION Per Serving: 247 calories; 5 grams protein; 49 grams carbohydrate; 4 grams fiber; 5 grams fat (3 grams saturated); 66 mg sodium

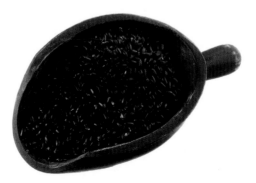

Mixed Fruit Smoothie

This fruit smoothie can be enjoyed for dessert or as a snack any time of day. *SERVES 2*

1¼ cups low-fat plain Greek yogurt

1½ cups frozen strawberries

¾ cup freshly squeezed orange juice

1 banana, cut into pieces

1 tablespoon agave nectar or honey

In a blender or food processor, add the yogurt, strawberries, orange juice, banana, and agave nectar. Puree until the strawberries are broken up and the smoothie is thoroughly blended, 30 seconds to 1 minute.

DO THE DASH   Smoothies are an excellent way to get the 4 to 6 fruit servings the DASH Diet recommends each day. Greek yogurt gives smoothies a creamy mouthfeel, plus plenty of beneficial probiotic bacteria, bone-building calcium, and protein.

SHOPPING TIP   Purchase only unsweetened yogurt for smoothies since you'll get plenty of sweetness from the fruit.

NUTRITION   Per Serving: 272 calories; 16 grams protein; 48 grams carbohydrate; 4 grams fiber; 3 grams fat (2 grams saturated); 51 mg sodium

Appendix

Techniques

A few basic techniques for prepping ingredients will make cooking fresh DASH-friendly meals even easier.

PEELING AN AVOCADO: Halve the avocado. Sink a sharp knife into the seed and pull it out. Holding one half of the avocado in the palm of your hand, insert a large spoon under the avocado flesh, next to the peel, and run it all around the avocado until you can lift the whole avocado half out of the peel.

PEELING A MANGO: Slice through the mango lengthwise, next to one side of the flat pit, and detach; repeat for the other side. Spoon out the flesh and chop or slice as needed.

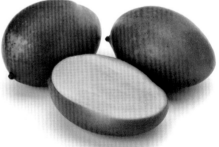

CLEANING LEEKS: Cut off the tough green leaves and the tip of the root end. Transfer to a bowl of cold water and swish the leeks vigorously to loosen the layers and remove any dirt. Leaf through the layers to see whether any soil remains. If needed, drain and repeat.

HULLING A TOMATO: Using a small paring knife, core the tomatoes, leaving a round opening. With a spoon or a melon baller, scoop out the insides, including the seeds. Don't scoop too close to the bottom or the tomatoes won't stay sturdy. Rinse the tomatoes with water and place them upside down to drain on a paper towel.

TRIMMING ASPARAGUS: The tough end of the asparagus needs to be removed before you eat it, but don't worry—Mother Nature makes it easy for you. Just bend the bottom part of the asparagus, about 1 to 2 inches from the bottom, and the stalk will snap at the point where tender meets tough. Go through a handful of asparagus at a time for ease.

CUTTING UP MEAT FOR STEW: Pull the meat apart at the seams, and trim the fat. Examine the pieces of meat to figure out the best way to go about cutting. Then cut the meat into 1½-inch cubes. Don't be tempted to cut smaller cubes; you need hefty pieces to prevent drying out.

SUPREMING CITRUS FRUIT: Use a serrated knife to slice off about ½ inch from the bottom of the fruit and the top. Place the fruit bottom-down on a work surface, and use the serrated knife to remove the peel and pith from the entire fruit. Over a bowl to catch the juice, use a paring knife to cut each segment from between the two membranes, dropping the segment into the bowl.

Conversions

Use this handy chart to scale any recipe to the size you need, or to determine quantities of unusual ingredients.

Measure	Equivalent	Metric
1 teaspoon	---	5 milliliters
1 tablespoon	3 teaspoons	14.8 milliliters
1 cup	16 tablespoons	236.8 milliliters
1 pint	2 cups	473.6 milliliters
1 quart	4 cups	947.2 milliliters
1 liter	4 cups + 3½ tablespoons	1000 milliliters
1 ounce (dry)	2 tablespoons	28.35 grams
1 pound	16 ounces	453.49 grams
2.21 pounds	35.3 ounces	1 kilogram
180°F / 350°F / 400°F	---	82°C / 180°C / 200°C

DASH Charts

Knowing how many servings of each food group you'll need per day, as well as what constitutes one serving in each category, will make following the DASH Diet guidelines a snap. The charts here and the guidelines on pages 9–10 will be useful for planning your DASH meals.

DASH Servings per Day		
Food Groups	*1,200 calories per day*	*2,000 calories per day*
Grains	3	4–5
Vegetables	4–5	5–6
Fruits	4	5–6
Low-fat and nonfat dairy	2–3	3
Lean meats, poultry, and fish	3–6 oz	6–7 oz
Nuts, seeds, and legumes	3–4 per week	4–5 per week
Fats and oils	2	3
Sweets and added sugars	0	fewer than 5 per week

General DASH Guidelines

Food Group	Daily Servings	Serving Sizes	Examples and Notes	Significance of Each Food Group to DASH
Grains	6–8	1 slice bread 1 oz dry cereal* ½ cup cooked rice, pasta, or cereal	100% whole wheat bread, pasta, English muffin, pita bread, bagel, cereal, grits, oatmeal, brown rice, unsalted pretzels, and popcorn	Major sources of energy and fiber
Vegetables	4–5	1 cup raw leafy vegetable ½ cup cut-up raw or cooked vegetable ½ cup vegetable juice	Broccoli, carrots, collard greens, eggplant, green beans, green peas, kale, lima beans, red potatoes, spinach, squash, sweet potatoes, tomatoes, zucchini	Rich sources of potassium, magnesium, fiber, and minerals
Fruits	4–5	1 medium whole fruit ¼ cup dried fruit ½ cup fresh, frozen, or canned fruit ½ cup fruit juice	Apples, apricots, bananas, berries, cherries, dates, grapes, oranges, grapefruit, grapefruit juice, mangoes, melons, nectarines, peaches, pears, pineapples, plums, raisins, strawberries, tangerines	Important sources of potassium, magnesium, fiber, and vitamins
Low-fat or nonfat dairy products	2–3	1 cup milk or yogurt ½ cup cottage cheese 1½ oz cheese	Nonfat (skim) or low-fat (1%) milk, low-fat cheese, low-fat plain regular, Greek, or frozen yogurt, low-fat cottage cheese	Major sources of calcium and protein
Lean meats, poultry, and fish	6 or fewer	1 oz cooked meat, poultry, or fish; 1 egg**	Lean meat, chicken, turkey, or fish; trim away visible fat; broil, roast, or poach; remove skin from poultry	Rich sources of protein and magnesium

General DASH Guidelines

Food Group	Daily Servings	Serving Sizes	Examples and Notes	Significance of Each Food Group to DASH
Nuts, seeds, and legumes	4–5 per week	⅓ cup or 1½ oz raw nuts 2 Tbsp nut butter 2 Tbsp or ½ oz raw seeds ½ cup cooked legumes	Raw, unsalted almonds, cashews, hazelnuts, peanuts, pecans, walnuts, sunflower seeds; peanut or almond butter; black, kidney, garbanzo, or pinto beans; lentils, split peas	Rich sources of energy, magnesium, protein, and fiber
Fats and oils***	2–3	1 tsp butter 1 tsp olive or vegetable oil 1 Tbsp mayonnaise 2 Tbsp salad dressing	Spreadable butter, canola, or olive oil; low-fat mayonnaise; light salad dressing	27% of calories as fat, including fat in or added to foods
Sweets and added sugars	5 or fewer per week	1 Tbsp sugar 1 Tbsp jelly or jam ½ cup sorbet or gelatin 1 cup lemonade	Fruit-flavored gelatin, hard candy, real fruit jelly or jam, maple syrup, sorbet and ices, sugar; avoid artificial sweeteners	Sweets should be low in fat, but not processed

* Serving sizes vary between ½ cup and 1¼ cups, depending on cereal type. Check the product's nutrition facts label and stick with 1 ounce.
** Since eggs are high in cholesterol, limit egg yolk intake to no more than 4 per week; 2 egg whites have the same protein content as 1 ounce of meat.
*** Fat content changes serving amount for fats and oils. For example: 1 tablespoon of regular salad dressing = 1 serving; 1 tablespoon of low-fat dressing = ½ serving; 1 tablespoon of nonfat dressing = 0 servings.
Chart reference: http://www.nhlbi.nih.gov/health/public/heart/hbp/dash/new_dash.pdf, modified by Ulysses

Recipe Index

About the Contributors

ANDREA LYNN is a food writer and recipe developer with a culinary arts degree from the Institute of Culinary Education. She has over a decade of experience as a writer and editor, including a multiyear stint as Senior Editor at *Chile Pepper* magazine. She continues to write and develop recipes for *Chile Pepper*, as well as the James Beard award–winning website *Serious Eats*. Andrea has worked in the kitchen of a three-star restaurant, as a personal chef, and as a culinary consultant. She is the author of *The I Love Trader Joe's College Cookbook* and *The Artisan Soda Workshop*. She lives in Astoria, New York. More information about Andrea is available at www.andrealynnfoodwriter.com.

MATT KADEY, author of *Muffin Tin Chef*, is a registered dietitian, freelance nutrition writer, recipe developer, and travel photographer based in Waterloo, Ontario, Canada. As a prolific magazine writer, his nutrition, recipe, and travel articles have appeared in dozens of prestigious publications, including *Men's Health, Alive, Women's Health, Shape, Prevention, Eating Well, Men's Journal, Vegetarian Times, Runner's World, Bicycling,* and *Fit Pregnancy*. As an avid cyclist, Matt has cycled and feasted his way through numerous countries, including Sri Lanka, New Zealand, Laos, Thailand, Cuba, Cambodia, Ireland, Ethiopia, Belize, and Jordan. He is also a former provincial mountain bike champion in his age category. You can find Matt at mattkadey.com or www.muffintinmania.com.